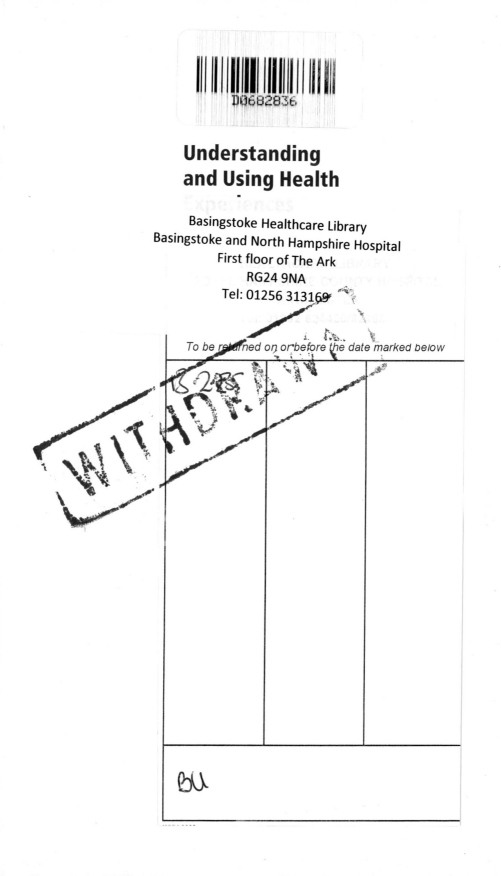
Understanding
and Using Health

Understanding and Using Health Experiences

Improving Patient Care

Edited by

Sue Ziebland
Reader in Qualitative Health Research and
Research Director of Health Experiences Research Group
Department of Primary Care Health Sciences
University of Oxford
Oxford, UK

Angela Coulter
Director of Global Initiatives
Informed Medical Decisions Foundation,
Boston, MA, USA and
Senior Research Scientist
Department of Public Health
University of Oxford
Oxford, UK

Joseph D. Calabrese
Head of Medical Anthropology
Department of Anthropology
University College London
London, UK

Louise Locock
Deputy Research Director
Health Experiences Research Group
Department of Primary Care Health Sciences
University of Oxford
Oxford, UK

OXFORD
UNIVERSITY PRESS

OXFORD
UNIVERSITY PRESS

Great Clarendon Street, Oxford OX2 6DP
United Kingdom

Oxford University Press is a department of the University of Oxford.
It furthers the University's objective of excellence in research, scholarship,
and education by publishing worldwide. Oxford is a registered trade mark of
Oxford University Press in the UK and in certain other countries

British Library Cataloguing in Publication Data
Data available

ISBN 978-0-19-966537-2

Oxford University Press makes no representation, express or implied, that the
drug dosages in this book are correct. Readers must therefore always check
the product information and clinical procedures with the most up-to-date
published product information and data sheets provided by the manufacturers
and the most recent codes of conduct and safety regulations. The authors and
the publishers do not accept responsibility or legal liability for any errors in the
text or for the misuse or misapplication of material in this work. Except where
otherwise stated, drug dosages and recommendations are for the non-pregnant
adult who is not breast-feeding.

Acknowledgements

The editors and authors would like to thank the following:

Our OUP editors, Caroline Smith and Nicola Wilson, for their help and support.

Vanessa Eade and Abi Eccles from the Health Experiences Research Group, for administrative assistance.

Green Templeton College, Oxford (especially Sir David Watson and Wendy Greenberg) for hosting the March 2011 Health Experiences Institute conference 'Do we know what patients want? Understanding and using patient experience' from which this book arose, and our first writing workshop.

Dr Phil Hammond for chairing the March conference with such insight and good humour.

The Community at the Abbey, Sutton Courtenay, for looking after us during our second writing workshop.

Dr Ann McPherson (1945–2011), for being the inspiration behind the Health Experiences Institute.

Contents

Contributors

Claire Anderson
Professor of Social Pharmacy
School of Pharmacy
University of Nottingham
Nottingham, UK

Joseph D. Calabrese
Head of Medical Anthropology
Department of Anthropology
University College
London, UK

Angela Coulter
Director of Global Initiatives
Informed Medical Decisions
Foundation
Boston, MA, USA and
Senior Research Scientist
Department of Public Health
University of Oxford
Oxford, UK

Ray Fitzpatrick
Professor of Public Health and
Primary Care
Department of Public Health
University of Oxford
Oxford, UK

Bob Gann
Director of Partnerships and
Engagement
NHS Choices
Department of Health
London, UK

Ruth Garside
Senior Lecturer in Evidence
Synthesis
European Centre for Environment
and Human Health
University of Exeter Medical School
University of Exeter
Exeter, UK

Chris Graham
Director of Survey Development
Picker Institute Europe
Oxford, UK

Trisha Greenhalgh
Professor of Primary Health Care
and Co-Director
Global Health, Policy and
Innovation Unit
Blizard Institute, Barts and
The London School of Medicine and
Dentistry
London, UK

Andrew Herxheimer
Clinical Pharmacologist
Emeritus Fellow
UK Cochrane Centre
Oxford, UK

Crispin Jenkinson
Director, Health Services Research
Unit and
Professor of Health Services
Research
Department of Public Health
University of Oxford
Oxford, UK

Jenny Kitzinger
Professor of Communications
Research
Director of the Health, Science, Risk,
Media Research Group
Cardiff University
Cardiff, UK

Louise Locock
Deputy Research Director
Health Experiences Research Group
Department of Primary
Care Health Sciences
University of Oxford
Oxford, UK

Fadhila Mazanderani
Lecturer in Sociology
School of Applied Social Sciences
Durham University
Durham, UK

John Powell
Senior Clinical Researcher
Department of Primary Care Health
Sciences
University of Oxford, Oxford and
Consultant Clinical Advisor
National Institute for Health and
Clinical Excellence
London, UK

Glenn Robert
Professor of Healthcare Quality and
Innovation
National Nursing Research Unit
King's College London
London, UK

Sara Ryan
Senior Research Lead
Health Experiences Research Group
University of Oxford
Oxford, UK

Fiona Stevenson
Senior Lecturer in Medical Sociology
Department of Primary Care and
Population Health
University College London
London, UK

Penny Woods
Chief Executive
British Lung Foundation
London, UK

Sue Ziebland
Reader in Qualitative Health
Research and
Research Director of Health
Experiences Research Group
Department of Primary Care Health
Sciences
University of Oxford
Oxford, UK

Chapter 1

Introduction

Sue Ziebland and Angela Coulter

Healthcare is a knowledge-based system. It draws on several different types of knowledge—scientific knowledge about biological processes, epidemiological knowledge about patterns of disease and risk factors, and clinical knowledge about how to treat medical problems. This book is concerned with a fourth type of knowledge that is equally important, but sometimes overlooked, namely how people experience health, illness, treatment, and the delivery of care. In putting the book together our aim was to introduce readers to the various ways in which people's experience of health and healthcare can be recorded, analysed, and, where necessary, improved.

Careful observation, measurement, recording, interpretation, and analysis of people's experiences can help us to appreciate what is working well in health-care, what needs to change, and how we might go about making improvements. The social scientists, health professionals, and policymakers who have contributed to this volume share a commitment to applied, multidisciplinary research. In this collection they describe a wide range of methods and types of data, showing what each adds to our understanding of health experiences. But this book is not 'just' an introduction to a range of methods for understanding health experiences; we also explain how the methods can be used to challenge and improve services.

Our approach is pluralist; we recognize that methods differ depending on the research questions, the intended application of the results, the interests and skills of the research team, the prospects for combining different methods, and the time available. Thus we include methods for collecting primary data using qualitative approaches (ethnography, observations, focus groups, storytelling, and narrative interviews) and quantitative methods (patient surveys and patient reported outcome measures (PROMs)). We also consider secondary sources which can provide valuable insight into health experiences: online blogs and communities, documentary analysis of adverse event reporting, and qualitative literature synthesis. Throughout, the authors give examples of how each method can be applied to monitor and improve crucial aspects of health services.

Understanding health experiences

Qualitative approaches to understanding health experiences include analysis of naturally occurring data as well as methods designed to generate people's accounts of their experiences through in-depth interviews, focus groups, and storytelling. These methods aim to find out what is important to the participants, including what meanings they attach to health and illness. There is of course a difference between what people *say* they do (for example, the accounts that they give in interviews, focus groups, or responses in face-to-face or self-completion questionnaire surveys) and what they *actually do* in natural settings. Behaviour in natural settings can be illuminated and interpreted through ethnographic observations and interaction analysis, although the impact of the research and the researcher on the setting always needs to be considered.

Ethnographic approaches (Chapter 3) require researchers to live or work within the community or setting, developing a rich understanding of practices by paying very close attention to what is happening around them. This type of study can illuminate how people understand, explain, and cope with their health problems. Stevenson shows how observations of patient–doctor interactions (Chapter 4), combined with detailed conversation and interaction analysis, give primacy to the detail of the interaction, revealing the features through which the work of the consultation is achieved. These features may not even be evident to the participants, yet analysis can reveal patterns that help explain how decisions are made and why actions are taken. The approach can be particularly useful for exploring verbal and non-verbal cues that may signify problems in communication.

Individual, narrative interviews have become popular because they encourage the participant to tell the story of what has happened to them in their own way, focusing on the issues that are important to them. Analysis needs to be rigorous and include anticipated and emergent themes as well as attending to how people construct their stories (Chapter 5). Some people can find it difficult to respond when invited by a researcher to recount their experiences in a one-to-one interview, but they may be less reticent in a discussion group of their peers. Focus groups rely on interactions between people with similar experiences in a facilitated discussion and have become widely used in designing services and interventions. Facilitation is a demanding task, requiring the researcher to ensure that different points of view are allowed to emerge and are respected by participants (Chapter 6). Storytelling groups (Chapter 7) are an interesting variant on group discussions; Trisha Greenhalgh demonstrates their value both as a source of data about how people perceive their health and as part of an intervention to support self-management in chronic illness.

Qualitative approaches such as these all rely on the skills of the researcher in conducting interviews or recording their observations. The approaches tend to be labour intensive with little division of labour and requiring lengthy and attentive analysis and interpretation. They are often regarded as reaching the parts of the experience that more structured methods cannot reach—yet are not designed to provide numerically representative estimates of prevalence. For this, and to identify patterns and correlations in the data, we need quantitative methods.

People's accounts of their experiences can be obtained on site at the point of contact with health services; several days, weeks, or months after an episode of treatment; or continuously, using diaries or similar methods.

Surveys using structured questionnaires are widely used as a quantitative measure of patients' experience (Chapter 9). They are designed to produce numerical data that can be analysed statistically and used to describe and compare results from a sample population and specific subgroups. Survey questions are usually 'closed', in that they offer a specific set of response options, and pre-coded, but it is also possible to include open-ended questions that can be coded at the data entry stage, or analysed using qualitative thematic methods (Garcia et al., 2004). Patient experience surveys use a variety of methods for collecting data, including face-to-face interviews, self-completion postal questionnaires, telephone interviews using live interviewers or automated interactive voice methods, web-based online questionnaires, and questions on hand-held portable devices, touch-screen kiosks, or bedside consoles.

In addition to gathering patients' views on the process of care, there is now considerable interest in investigating their reports of health outcomes. PROMs are increasingly used in quantitative research, especially in randomized trials that evaluate the effects of treatment and for monitoring performance in different settings (Chapter 8). These types of measures enable assessment of the effects of medical interventions on patients' physical and emotional functioning and quality of life. There is now a huge array of measures, most of which have been designed for specific purposes or patient groups. The best of these probably get closer to what is important to patients than many of the clinical indicators that have been measured traditionally, leading to interest in the potential for PROMS to be used in routine clinical practice.

Secondary sources

As well as data that is generated through observation, interviews, groups, and surveys there are other sources of information that can provide highly informative data about health experiences. The Internet is foremost among these; in

Chapter 10 Mazanderani and Powell discuss blogs, forums, chat rooms, feedback, and social networking sites as a resource for exploring 'naturally occurring' health experiences. There are ethical issues involved in collecting data from these sources but many researchers conclude that if the material is published in the public domain it should be treated in a similar way to other media sources. Quantitative or qualitative analytic approaches can be used for media content analysis. In Chapter 12 Anderson and Herxheimer consider the potential for documentary analysis of patients' reports of adverse drug reactions to support pharmacovigilance. Post-marketing surveillance and adverse event reporting is crucial for understanding risks associated with the use of medicines, and systems have been established in a number of countries to enable patients to provide direct reports of adverse reactions to drugs. Comparison of these reports with those from professionals shows that patients' accounts can add a new and potentially rich source of knowledge about the effects of medicines, including previously unrecognized side effects and risks.

Systematic reviews of randomized controlled trials and other types of quantitative study form the bedrock of evidence-based medicine. Qualitative data on health and illness experiences have been challenging to locate and synthesize but as Garside shows in Chapter 11 there are now clearly established methods for undertaking qualitative synthesis. The methods are increasingly used to inform the development of National Institute for Health and Clinical Excellence (NICE) clinical guidelines, especially in the field of public health.

Ryan (Chapter 13) reminds us about the importance of inclusivity at all stages of the research process from design and ethics clearance through to reporting the finding and offers examples of good practice. Non-traditional methods of data collection, using pictures, stories, or drama, may help to ensure that the views and experiences of those in 'hard-to-reach' or 'seldom-heard' groups are not excluded from research, and therefore from our understanding of what is important to a wide range of patients and the public.

Using research on health experiences

The chapters include numerous examples of how health experiences can be applied to improve services. Chapter 2 traces the development of this field of research and the growing interest of policymakers in techniques for ensuring that healthcare systems are responsive to the needs and concerns of the patients they serve. Coulter describes how monitoring patients' experiences came to be seen as a crucial element in quality assurance, helping to redress the imbalance between the technological focus of much of modern medical care and the interpersonal aspects that are so important to patients. Some seminal studies are briefly outlined and the chapter explains how the knowledge gained from studies of health and illness experiences can be used to transform the quality of care. In Chapter 14 Robert shows how mixed methods, including narrative interviews about healthcare experiences, can be used to prompt improvements to services through experience based co-design. This form of participatory action research brings staff and users together to share their experiences of giving and receiving healthcare. Participants work together to re-design services building on their shared knowledge of the strengths and weaknesses of the existing system. This approach also draws on user-centred design, learning theory, and expert facilitation to encourage systematic and sustainable improvements.

In the final chapter, Gann returns to the policy theme, illustrating how this knowledge is now considered essential for quality improvement, accountability, and for helping patients make informed choices about their treatment and care. Whereas large-scale surveys were once considered the only reliable way to monitor the quality of care from the patient's perspective, the Internet has opened up a variety of new ways of obtaining, providing, and sharing information on patients' experiences and preferences. The emphasis now is on plurality and experimentation, drawing on the rich tapestry of methods outlined in this book to extend and deepen our understanding of what matters to those who use healthcare services.

Reference

Garcia, J., Evans, J., and Reshaw, M. (2004). Is there anything else you would like to tell us? Methodologica: issues in the use of free-text comments from postal surveys. *Quality and Quantity*, 38, 113–25.

Chapter 2

Understanding the experience of illness and treatment

Angela Coulter

> To study the phenomenon of diseases without books
> is to sail an uncharted sea, while to study books
> without patients is not to go to sea at all.
> William Osler (1849–1919)

Introduction

There is an unfortunate paradox at the centre of modern medical care. As medical knowledge has advanced, offering considerable benefits in terms of more effective treatments, so healthcare delivery has become progressively more complex, fragmented, and difficult to manage. William Osler, widely recognized as the father of modern medicine, stressed the need to listen to patients and learn from their experiences, but scientific developments have tended to inhibit the extent to which this good advice is acted upon. Rapid progress in science-based medicine and the resulting proliferation of technologies and treatments has distracted attention from the human experience of being ill and the search for cures has overshadowed the important business of caring for people.

Talcott Parsons described illness as 'a state of disturbance in the "normal" functioning of the total human individual, including both the state of the organism as a biological system and of his personal and social adjustment. It is thus partly biologically and partly socially defined' (Parsons, 1951, p. 431). Since then, various commentators, mostly social and behavioural scientists, have criticized medical science for focusing its efforts on understanding and manipulating the biological system while paying only cursory attention to the personal and social aspects. It is certainly true that the emphasis on biological science has reaped considerable rewards. Many conditions that could not be treated at the time Parsons was writing can now be dealt with effectively, leading to significant gains in length and quality of life. But the clamour from patients complaining of difficulties in navigating the system, of uncommunicative staff, and lack of practical and emotional support grows ever louder. The technological advances have come at a cost, namely the tendency of biomedical science to marginalize and undervalue the 'softer' notions of caring, compassion, and respectful delivery of healthcare. It is not that health professionals don't care. On the contrary, most people who choose to work in healthcare are motivated by a strong desire to relieve suffering, but the very complexity of modern health systems means they are required to focus on protocols, tasks, and techniques that can get in the way of responding appropriately to patients' personal and emotional needs.

Historical context

It was not only social scientists who called for more attention to be paid to patients' experiences; influential clinicians and patient organizations also played leading roles. Roy Porter traced the origins of today's patient groups to 'the 1960s popular counter-culture backlash against scientific and technological arrogance' (Porter, 2003). Some of these groups had their origins in the women's movement; stimulated by feminist writings that were critical of the medical profession's domination of healthcare, they promoted mutual self-help and demystification of medical knowledge. Others established single-issue campaigns, like the National Association for the Welfare of Children in Hospital, founded in 1961, which mobilized public opinion against the then common practice of separating children from their parents during long hospital stays. The 1980s saw rapid growth in the number of patient organizations and collectively they began to wield political influence. Some of these groups were developed and actively supported by health professionals; for example, patient partnership groups in general practice were first established in the 1970s.

The government responded to this increase in patient activism with various policy initiatives designed to strengthen the voice of patients, including the establishment in 1974 of 182 local Community Health Councils to represent patients' interests. Following the 1979 general election when Margaret Thatcher's government came to power, the emphasis switched from social rights towards a more consumerist approach (Hogg, 2009). New ideas about public management were promoted and the first steps were taken towards introducing an internal market based on competition and patient choice into the healthcare system. The regulations about general practice registration were amended to make it easier for patients to vote with their feet if they were unhappy with their care. This period also saw the first attempts to reduce dependence on healthcare resources by strengthening prevention and encouraging self-care. The policy focus on patient-centred care that gathered strength from the 1980s onwards was an attempt to restore the equilibrium between curing and caring, recognizing and strengthening the patient's role as a co-producer of health (Coulter, 2011).

The Labour government that came to power in 1997 retained and strengthened many of these innovations, despite its initial opposition to them. This period also saw the development of the national patient survey programme, another attempt to use the voice of the patient to stimulate quality improvements in healthcare. A further important breakthrough came in 2008 when it was officially acknowledged that patients' experiences were as important as clinical effectiveness and safety in defining high-quality care (Secretary of State for Health, 2008). This was followed by the NHS Constitution, setting out the standards and rights that a patient could expect (Department of Health, 2009), and a renewed commitment to measure performance systematically, with a special focus on health outcomes and patients' experience (Department of Health, 2010). At the time of writing we have a coalition government in England that has embarked on yet another round of reforms, with the stated commitment that 'patients will be at the heart of everything we do' (Secretary of State for Health, 2010). Healthcare commissioners and provider organizations are expected to build their quality assurance systems on a detailed understanding of patients' experience of care, using every feasible opportunity to obtain and take note of service users' accounts of 'how it was' for them.

Seeing things through patients' eyes

The renewed focus on understanding patients' experience constitutes an attempt to address the imbalance of knowledge, skills, and research effort with the aim of making care more patient-centred. But these ideas did not arise from nowhere. There is a long and distinguished tradition of empirical research and theoretical analysis to draw on, including many different methods and techniques for gathering and analysing health experiences. Each of the following chapters looks at a specific approach in some detail, exploring its strengths and limitations and providing examples of how it has been applied. But first we should briefly look at what distinguishes the focus on illness experiences from a focus on disease.

Two psychoanalysts working in Britain in the 1950s, Michael and Enid Balint, are credited with first developing the notion that care could be either 'illness-oriented' or 'patient-centred' (Balint, 1969). In their formulation, patient-centred medicine meant understanding the patient as a unique human being and being concerned with the whole person, mind as well as body. They suggested that doctors should listen carefully to patients and be willing to discuss personal or emotional issues that go beyond the ostensible reason for consultation, responding flexibly as required. They established group seminars for general practitioners to explore the emotional content of the doctor–patient relationship and Balint groups continue to meet in many countries to the present day.

The term 'patient-centred care' is now widely used but there is often confusion about what it means (Mead and Bower, 2000; Holmstrom and Roing, 2010). Most writers agree that it is multidimensional, but there is considerable debate about which dimensions are the most important (Entwistle et al., 2012). Mead and Bower reviewed the literature on patient-centredness and its measurement and identified five distinct dimensions:

1. A biopsychosocial perspective, i.e. concern with the 'non-medical' aspects of care (similar to the Balints' definition of the concept)

2. A biographical focus on the 'patient as person'

3. An egalitarian sharing of power and responsibility

4. A therapeutic alliance based on the personal relationship between doctor and patient

5. A focus on the qualities of the 'doctor [or nurse] as person' (Mead and Bower, 2000).

This is very different from the concerns of clinical research with its focus on understanding biological signs and bodily malfunctions and testing ways of modifying these. It has somewhat more in common with epidemiology, where the aim is to understand the causes of disease by studying its distribution in populations, taking account of the socio-economic factors that influence disease incidence and prevalence. But epidemiologists do not usually concern themselves with people's emotional and practical responses to illness, which is central to our focus here.

Why does this matter? The scientific, clinical, and epidemiological knowledge base is clearly crucial for effective healthcare, but it is also important that healthcare systems respond sensitively to the needs and concerns of health service users. This cannot be done effectively without a deep knowledge of their perspective. While clinicians may feel they have a good understanding of their patients' needs, evidence suggests there is often a mismatch between the views and concerns of professionals and those of their patients (Rozenblum et al., 2011; Mulley et al., 2012). Furthermore, a growing body of evidence suggests that patient-centred care can lead to improved health outcomes. For example, studies have shown that patients whose treatment is deemed patient-centred are more likely to trust their clinicians (Keating et al., 2002), more likely to adhere to treatment recommendations (Haynes et al., 2008), and less likely to die following a major event such as acute myocardial infarction (Glickman et al., 2010; Meterko et al., 2010). It may also help to reduce dependence on medical interventions or invasive treatments, leading to reductions in healthcare utilization and costs (Stewart et al., 2000; Little et al., 2001; Bertakis and Azari, 2011; Stacey et al., 2011). Quite why a patient-centred approach should have these effects is not entirely understood, but it seems likely that improved understanding of their condition enhances patients' ability to look after themselves; that those who are more involved in decisions have greater commitment to agreed treatment plans making it more likely that they will adhere to clinical recommendations; and attention to the patient's social context may help to enhance family and social support, leading to improvements in emotional well-being (Street et al., 2009). Also, an association has been noted between patient satisfaction and technical quality, underlining the fact that the best providers manage to combine technical excellence and good interpersonal skills to offer truly patient-centred care (Isaac et al., 2010).

Influential studies of illness experiences

During the latter part of the 20th century, several prominent American and British researchers made detailed studies of patients' experience of being ill and receiving treatment that led to calls for radical change. Especially influential were Erving Goffman (Goffman, 1961), Ann Cartwright (Cartwright, 1967), David Tuckett (Tuckett et al., 1985), Arthur Kleinman (Kleinman, 1988), and Paul Cleary (Cleary et al., 1991). Goffman and Kleinman used ethnographic methods to study doctor–patient interactions, Cartwright and Cleary primarily used patient surveys, while Tuckett and his colleagues used a combination of qualitative and quantitative methods. These studies provided important insights, some of which had a profound influence on subsequent policy developments. Goffman's study of the lives of patients in a psychiatric hospital was a landmark publication that drew attention to the negative consequences of institutionalization and helped to change public attitudes to long-term mental health care (Goffman, 1961). Cartwright and Tuckett studied the experience of patients in British general practices, pointing to communication and organizational failures and their consequences (Cartwright and Anderson, 1981; Tuckett et al., 1985). Kleinman's study of the illness experience of people with chronic conditions led to a critique of postgraduate medical training programmes which, he argued, encouraged behaviours that were 'antithetical to the humane care of patients' (Kleinman, 1988) (p. 257). Kleinman urged medical educators to 'make the patient's and family's narrative of the illness experience more central in the educational process' (p.255).

Another important development in the understanding of patients' experience occurred in 1986 with the launch of the Picker/Commonwealth Patient-Centred Care Program (Beatrice et al., 1998). This substantial grant programme sought to explore how patients experience care in medical settings, the constraints and opportunities faced by those wanting to improve care quality, and what health professionals could do to enhance patient-centred care. This led to the development of a widely-used suite of surveys to measure patients' experience, the establishment of a charitable institution, the Picker Institute, with a remit to research and improve patient care, and a book, *Through the Patient's Eyes* (Gerteis et al., 1993), that summarized the findings of the research programme and presented a practical framework to help managers and providers improve their ability to meet patients' needs. The framework eventually resurfaced in an important US report on healthcare quality, *Crossing the Quality Chasm* (Institute of Medicine, 2001), that was influential on both sides of the Atlantic. Government, health authority, or insurer-sponsored patient surveys are now conducted regularly in many countries, including Canada, Denmark, England, Ireland, Japan, Hong Kong, Netherlands, Norway, Scotland, Sweden, Turkey, and the USA (Garratt et al., 2008).

While patient surveys are now seen as essential for monitoring and improving the quality of healthcare, more detailed narratives of patients' experiences have been used as a means of motivating clinicians to review and change their practice. Two highly talented medical writers and commentators, Don Berwick and Atul Gawande, epitomize this approach. Neither of them would claim to be professional ethnographers like Goffman or Kleinman, but both have used patients' stories to good effect to illustrate particular issues in relation to the quality of care. Often drawing on the experience of family, friends, or their own patients, these medical doctors know how to grab the attention of professional and public readers to illustrate serious points. For example, in a much-quoted article Berwick used an account of how clinical staff refused to allow him to accompany a close friend while she was undergoing cardiac catheterization as an arresting prelude to a discussion about patient-centredness and the abuse of professional power (Berwick, 2009). Gawande, a surgeon who writes a regular column in *The New Yorker*, has written numerous accounts of patients' and clinicians' experiences as part of his campaign to improve standards of surgical care (Gawande, 2009). These writers know that engaging readers emotionally can be more powerful than overwhelming them with facts—stories often trump data when there is a need to motivate people to think and act differently (see Chapter 14 for an account of how empathy and understanding can form an important component of quality improvement efforts).

Both qualitative (narrative and observation) and quantitative (survey) approaches have been used to increase understanding of the patient's perspective, but often a combination of methods is preferable. Selecting a method that is appropriate for the purpose for which it is needed must be done with care. Patients' stories and observations can be a particularly useful catalyst for change, but surveys are usually essential for monitoring trends and outcomes. As the following chapters make clear, each approach has strengths and weaknesses that must be taken into account.

From knowledge to action

Anyone who asks patients to devote time to talking about their experiences or completing a questionnaire ought to have a clear idea of what they will do with the data. It is unethical to request this type of participation for no good reason. In addition to the academic commitment to expanding knowledge, there are various reasons why it may be important to improve understanding of patients' experiences (Coulter et al., 2009). These include:

- Helping professionals reflect on their own and their team's practice
- Tackling specific problems in care delivery
- Informing continuous improvement and redesign of services
- Facilitating benchmarking between services and organizations
- Comparing organizations for performance assessment purposes
- Monitoring the impact of any changes
- Informing patients about care pathways
- Informing referring clinicians about the quality of services
- Informing commissioners and patients about the quality of services
- Helping patients choose high-quality providers
- Enabling public accountability.

If researchers are to contribute to these goals, they must ensure that their findings are accessible to practitioners, patients, and members of the public, as well as fellow researchers. This is likely to require the use of a variety of dissemination methods, based on a careful analysis of contexts and target audiences. Modes of dissemination might include brief articles, oral presentations, web-based summaries and indicators, handbooks and guidance, policy or procedure recommendations, information or communication tools, and training materials or courses.

Strategies for translating new knowledge into action should be based on an understanding of the factors that influence the likelihood of change. At the organizational level these may include the quality and commitment of the leadership, clarity of goals, identification of dedicated champions, active engagement of patients and families, staff skills, training and capacity, and availability of resources, in addition to the quality and depth of understanding of the patient's perspective (Davies et al., 2008; Luxford et al., 2011). For individuals it may depend on their knowledge, confidence, and commitment and the extent to which they feel empowered to make changes in their working practices. It is also important to understand possible barriers and constraints, including a widespread perception that improving patients' experience is not as high a priority on the national policy agenda as patient safety or sound financial management, the challenge of coping with multiple competing pressures, a feeling of being hidebound by policies, procedures, and regulatory requirements, the lack of a dedicated team to focus on quality improvement, and negative or defensive reactions from staff when patients are critical of their care (Coulter, 2012).

If we believe that patients' experiences are a key component of healthcare quality, then we must try to understand those experiences by careful observation, measurement, and analysis. We need to determine what is working well and should therefore be preserved, and what needs to be improved, and we must then act on this knowledge. To misquote Karl Marx, interpreting the world is never enough; the point is to change it.

Further reading

Ballatt, J. and Campling, P. (2011). *Intelligent kindness: Reforming the culture of healthcare.* London: Royal College of Psychiatrists.

Frampton, S.B. (2009). *Putting patients first: Best practices in patient-centred care.* San Francisco, CA: Jossey-Bass.

Gerteis, M., *et al.* (1993). *Through the patient's eyes: Understanding and promoting patient-centered care.* San Francisco, CA: Jossey-Bass.

Katz, J. (2002). *The silent world of doctor and patient.* Baltimore, MD: Johns Hopkins University Press.

Kleinman, A. (1988). *The illness narratives: Suffering, healing and the human condition.* New York, NY: Basic Books.

References

Balint, E. (1969). The possibilities of patient-centred medicine. *Journal of the College of General Practitioners, 17,* 269–76.

Beatrice, D.F., Thomas, C.P., and Biles, B. (1998). Grant making with an impact: the Picker/Commonwealth patient-centred care program. *Health Affairs, 17,* 236–44.

Bertakis, K.D. and Azari, R. (2011). Patient-centered care is associated with decreased health care utilization. *Journal of the American Board of Family Medicine, 24,* 229–39.

Berwick, D.M. (2009). What 'patient-centered' should mean: confessions of an extremist. *Health Affairs (Millwood), 28,* 555–65.

Cartwright, A. (1967). *Patients and their doctors.* London: Routledge and Kegan Paul.

Cartwright, A. and Anderson, R. (1981). *General practice revisited: A second study of patients and their doctors.* London: Routledge.

Cleary, P.D., *et al.* (1991). Patients evaluate their hospital care: a national survey. *Health Affairs, 10,* 254–67.

Coulter, A. (2011). *Engaging patients in healthcare.* Maidenhead: Open University Press.

Coulter, A. (2012). *Leadership for patient engagement.* London: King's Fund.

Coulter, A., Fitzpatrick, R., and Cornwell, J. (2009). *Measures of patients' experience in hospital: Purpose, methods and uses.* London: King's Fund.

Davies, E., *et al.* (2008). Evaluating the use of a modified CAHPS survey to support improvements in patient-centred care: lessons from a quality improvement collaborative. *Health Expectations, 11,* 160–76.

Department of Health (2009). *The NHS Constitution.* London: Department of Health.

Department of Health (2010). *The NHS Outcomes Framework 2011/12.* London: Department of Health.

Entwistle, V., *et al.* (2012). Which experiences of health care delivery matter to service users and why? A critical interpretive synthesis and conceptual map. *Journal of Health Services Research & Policy, 17,* 70–8.

Garratt, A.M., Solheim, E., and Danielsen, K. (2008). *National and cross-national surveys of patient experiences: A structured review.* Oslo: Norwegian Knowledge Centre for the Health Services.

Gawande, A. (2009). *The checklist manifesto: How to get things right.* London: Profile Books.

Gerteis, M., *et al.* (1993). *Through the patient's eyes: Understanding and promoting patient-centred care.* San Francisco, CA: Jossey Bass.

Glickman, S.W., *et al.* (2010). Patient satisfaction and its relationship with clinical quality and inpatient mortality in acute myocardial infarction. *Circulation: Cardiovascular Quality and Outcomes, 3,* 188–95.

Goffman, E. (1961). *Asylums: Essays on the social situation of mental patients and other inmates.* New York, NY: Anchor Books.

Haynes, R.B., *et al.* (2008). Interventions for enhancing medication adherence. *Cochrane Database of Systematic Reveiws, 2,* CD000011.

Hogg, C. (2009). *Citizens, consumers and the NHS: Capturing voices.* Basingstoke: Palgrave Macmillan.

Holmstrom, I. and Roing, M. (2010). The relation between patient-centeredness and patient empowerment: a discussion on concepts. *Patient Education and Counseling*, *79*, 167–72.

Institute of Medicine. (2001). *Crossing the quality chasm: A new health system for the 21st century*. Washington, DC: National Academy Press.

Isaac, T., *et al.* (2010). The relationship between patients' perception of care and measures of hospital quality and safety. *Health Services Research*, *45*, 1024–40.

Keating, N.L., *et al.* (2002). How are patients' specific ambulatory care experiences related to trust, satisfaction, and considering changing physicians? *Journal of General Internal Medicine*, *17*, 29–39.

Kleinman, A. (1988). *The illness narratives: Suffering, healing and the human Condition*. New York, NY: Basic Books.

Little, P., *et al.* (2001). Observational study of effect of patient centredness and positive approach on outcomes of general practice consultations. *British Medical Journal*, *323*, 908–11.

Luxford, K., *et al.* (2011). Promoting patient-centered care: a qualitative study of facilitators and barriers in healthcare organizations with a reputation for improving the patient experience. *International Journal for Quality in Health Care*, *23*, 510–15.

Mead, N. and Bower, P. (2000). Patient-centredness: a conceptual framework and review of the empirical literature. *Social Science and Medicine*, *51*, 1087–110.

Meterko, M., *et al.* (2010). Mortality among patients with acute myocardial infarction: the influences of patient-centered care and evidence-based medicine. *Health Services Research*, *45*, 1188–204.

Mulley, A., Trimble, C., and Elwyn, G. (2012). *Patients' preferences matter*. London: King's Fund.

Parsons, T. (1951). *The social system*. Glencoe, IL: Free Press.

Porter, R. (2003). *Blood and guts: A short history of medicine*. London: Penguin Books.

Rozenblum, R., *et al.* (2011). Uncovering the blind spot of patient satisfaction: an international survey. *British Medical Journal Quality and Safety*, *20*, 959–65.

Secretary of State for Health. (2008). *High quality care for all: NHS next stage review final report*. London: Department of Health.

Secretary of State for Health. (2010). *Equity and excellence: Liberating the NHS*. London: The Stationery Office.

Stacey, D., *et al.* (2011). Decision aids for people facing health treatment or screening decisions. *Cochrane Database of Systematic Reviews*, *10*, CD001431.

Stewart, M., *et al.* (2000). The impact of patient-centered care on outcomes. *Journal of Family Practice*, *49*, 796–804.

Street, R.L., *et al.* (2009). How does communication heal? Pathways linking clinician-patient communication to health outcomes. *Patient Education and Counseling*, *74*, 295–301.

Tuckett, D., *et al.* (1985). *Meetings between experts*. London: Tavistock.

Chapter 3

Ethnographic approaches to health experiences research

Joseph D. Calabrese

Ethnographers studying health experiences immerse themselves in social contexts of illness and treatment for prolonged periods of fieldwork to collect descriptive data and form an understanding of local culture and embodied experience. They pay very close attention to the experiences and interpretations of members of the group in question, studied in their natural context, and typically go for a depth of understanding (a small sample size studied intensively) rather than large sample sizes and attempts at statistical generalizability. The most distinctive method that ethnographers use is participant observation, which involves becoming a part of the everyday life and activities of a particular community, forming ongoing personal relationships, and observing social interaction and community life from the inside.

Ethnographic studies typically use open-ended, and often informal, narrative interviewing of social actors to learn about their personal experiences, their views on social practices, and their broader perceptions and opinions (see Chapter 5). Prolonged participant observation also reveals what people actually do in their activities and the nature of their social contexts. Ethnographers consider it important to study what people actually do as well as what they say they do, which may be different. Ethnographic research may be overt or covert. However, covert ethnography (in which subjects are not informed about the research) raises many difficult ethical questions and it is increasingly difficult to make an ethical case and gain ethical clearance for such studies. More often, the ethnographer forms a relationship with a gate-keeper (a local person in a position to facilitate or prevent the research) to gain access to the field site.

In comparison to other approaches to health experiences, ethnographic approaches to observation and interviewing emphasize a detailed understanding of the *social* or collective aspects of experience in addition to personal aspects, as in the focus of Kleinman and colleagues (1997) on 'social suffering'. Personal experiences of health and illness are thus contextualized in terms of social history, social relations, socially-transmitted understandings and attitudes (e.g. stigma), economic structures and inequalities, power relations, and moral orientations. As Good (1994, p. 5) states, medical language is 'a rich cultural language' that reflects deep moral concerns as well as medical realities.

Ethnographic observations, when recorded in writing, as in a field diary, are called field notes (Sanjek, 1990). These field notes help ethnographers construct 'thick descriptions' of their field sites, describing interactions and events in minute detail, but also contextualizing them in terms of the local webs of cultural meaning (Geertz, 1973). Ethnographers also record and transcribe interviews when they can, which, along with field notes, provide raw material for analysis. Analytical methods in ethnography are usually inductive, aimed at identifying patterns in the data—such as cultural themes—rather than imposing a priori concepts. Ethnographers most often stress qualitative forms of data but they may also use multiple methods to triangulate, generating rich and diverse bodies of data that may include measurements and numbers as well as narrative data, visual data, and artefacts.

Whatever the methods used, the ethnographer is the main research instrument and subjectivity is inevitable. Subjectivity refers to the unique perspective and personal identity of the ethnographer, including such things as the ethnographer's personal history, cultural assumptions, theoretical orientations, and values, which may bias ethnographic description if not examined and managed. The characteristic response of contemporary ethnographers to subjectivity is to adopt a reflexive understanding, exploring one's cultural and personal background and potential biases, and to include descriptions of one's identity and role in the field. 'Objective' description completely detached from a particular ethnographer's subjectivity is impossible. But a self-reflective awareness of one's personal identity helps the ethnographer take his or her subjectivity into account. Conveying this awareness to the readers also allows them to better evaluate the information presented.

Medical anthropology and the sociocultural contexts of health and illness

Ethnographic approaches were first developed in anthropology (Malinowski, 1922; Mead, 1928) and generally reflect the orientations of this discipline. Ethnographic approaches have also heavily influenced other disciplines, as in the Chicago School of Sociology (Whyte, 1943/1993). Anthropology takes a very broad view of humans as a species that developed in Africa and spread to occupy ecological niches from the Arctic to the deep desert. The cultural diversity resulting from these migrations and local paths of development over millennia included not only the development of warm clothing, agriculture, and mutually unintelligible languages but also many different understandings of health and illness. Human societies have developed diverse ways of conceptualizing and sustaining health associated with particular social histories and contexts. In many cases, similar challenges were addressed using different local methods and these choices became 'common sense' in the local culture. It is important to add here that this is as true for contemporary British or American society as it is for other societies: people tend to view the particular historical choices of their own society as common sense or 'normal' even when other choices are equally plausible or healthy.

Early applications of ethnographic data to health issues often took place in the context of colonial medicine, in which the goal was typically that of maintaining a healthy colonial workforce (Rubinstein and Lane, 1990). This work contributed to the development of medical anthropology, which came to focus on the diverse range of human approaches to illness and healing. Some important ethnographic works in this tradition include Devereux's (1961) work on psychiatric knowledge, psychic disturbances, and suicide among the Mohave Indians; Good's (1977) study of semantic networks surrounding illness in Iran; and Kleinman's (1980) study of doctor–patient relations in Taiwan.

As medical anthropology developed a broad comparative focus, and as the culture concept broadened to encompass not only the culture of those from exotic societies but humans generally, the ethnographic lens was increasingly applied to analysis of the ethnographer's own society and its cultural orientations. This resulted in ethnographers studying hospitals, asylums, and other medical settings in industrialized Western contexts.

The development of clinical ethnography

Several contemporary ethnographers of clinical topics and settings (Good et al., 1982; Herdt and Stoller, 1990; Luhrmann, 2000; Calabrese, in press) have used the term 'clinical ethnography' to describe their approach. I define clinical ethnography as culturally- and clinically-informed self-reflective immersion in local worlds of suffering, healing, and well-being to produce data that is of clinical as well as anthropological value.

The term 'clinical ethnography' emphasizes the clinical utility of ethnographic data. As Good and colleagues (1982, p. 282) state, in a clinical ethnography approach, ethnographic observations can be considered 'a central component of the therapeutic work' rather than of exclusively anthropological interest. Clinical ethnography also implies that the ethnography will be informed by a competent understanding of the clinical domain in question and may even involve the use of clinical methods or clinical practice in the field. Examples of the use of clinical methods in ethnography include Herdt and Stoller's (1990) use of psychoanalytic modes of reflexivity in interviews with the Sambia of New Guinea and my own application of local clinical practice as a mode of participant observation in Native American communities (Calabrese, 2008, in press). This method does not require full clinical training but the ethnographer must not be completely naïve about the standard clinical understandings of a particular domain of health. For example, an ethnographer studying mental illness should be familiar with the major categories of symptoms that may be experienced in these disorders (e.g. psychotic auditory hallucinations, intense anxiety, or suicidal thoughts).

Though having relevant clinical knowledge is important, an open-minded, self-reflective approach is essential, accepting that the clinical wisdom of the ethnographer's home society may be seen as deriving from that society's particular cultural orientations and norms, which may be irrelevant to other societies or even to certain patients or clinical staff in one's own society. Good (1994) argues effectively that human medical knowledge tends to reflect cultural and moral ideologies of the society in question. As such, he suggests that:

> anthropologists interested in the comparative study of illness and its treatment do well to move dialectically between a critical analysis of biomedical categories and knowledge, on the one hand, and operationalizations of such categories for the purposes of comparative, cross-cultural analysis, on the other (Good, 1994, p.168).

Just as clinical ethnographers must avoid being naïve about clinical matters, they should also avoid being naïve about the social and cultural diversity of the human species. The ethnographer should have some idea of the range of variation in human responses to illness, healing, and 'the normal'. When interviewing culturally diverse patients, for example, they should be aware that illness may be explained in terms of soul loss, spirit possession, witchcraft, punishment by a deity, or an imbalance of hotness and coldness in the body. These are all common explanations for illness cross-culturally.

Early examples of ethnographers aiming to closely observe and even approximate the perspectives of insiders in clinical settings include Caudill and Goffman, who both did extended fieldwork in psychiatric hospitals. Caudill (1958) studied the Yale Psychiatric Institute, initially in the role of a pseudo-patient for two months and then as an unconcealed field researcher focusing on social relations at the hospital. Goffman (1961) spent a year at a psychiatric hospital in Washington, DC, posing as a staff member and gathering data on hidden aspects of the lived experiences of mental patients.

Clinical ethnographers have conducted participant observation studies of a variety of other clinically-relevant topics, including patients' explanations of high blood pressure (Garro, 1988), experiences of patients with AIDS in Brazil (Biehl, 2006), surgical rituals and the culture of surgeons (Katz, 1981), experiences of homeless people with mental illness (Desjarlais, 1994), experiences of medical training at Harvard Medical School (Good and Good, 1993), and mental illness among immigrants in the context of racism and prejudice in the UK (Littlewood and Lipsedge, 1982). Mattingly (1994) worked closely with occupational therapists and studied the ways they used their interactions with patients to develop therapeutic plot structures supporting the treatment process. Anthropologist Susan DiGiacomo (1987) was diagnosed with Hodgkin's lymphoma during her dissertation research and thickly described her own illness and treatment, including her feelings of being an ignored bystander as the medical system conducted its war directly against her disease. Perhaps the best known experience-focused clinical ethnographer currently is Paul Farmer (2004), whose writings on Haiti tack back and forth between (1) thick descriptions of the experiences of suffering patients and his own experiences of challenging contexts of healthcare delivery and (2) the more global levels of inequality and structural violence, making clear the links between the local and the transnational.

What ethnography can contribute to understanding and improving health experiences

Among the most important strengths of ethnography as an approach to health experiences research is that it reduces the likelihood that important medical or policy decisions 'will be based on stereotypic oversimplifications and/or insufficient information' (Koehn, 2006). Approaches such as structured surveys collect data using questionnaires or interview schedules with pre-specified response categories (see Chapter 9). With qualitative methods, such as the ethnographic approach, we can discover some new, emergent information that we had not anticipated. In addition, if we are interviewing people in their homes or places of work, we are exploring health experiences in their natural contexts and we can learn important things from paying attention to those contexts.

Clinical ethnography not only contributes to medical anthropology as a distinct domain of anthropological understanding; it also provides crucial information to health systems. Ethnographic studies of patient experiences can clarify how patients interpret and implement medical directives and such studies can identify areas of patient dissatisfaction, important misunderstandings, and barriers to patient adherence and treatment seeking, such as inability to afford medication, cultural and language differences, distrust of the medical system, past negative experiences, and stigma. If patient motivation and likelihood to adhere to medical instructions are not taken into account, there may be disastrous results beyond poor outcomes for the individual patient, such as when sporadic adherence to medication regimens produces treatment-resistant forms of infectious diseases. Health experiences, of the type studied by clinical ethnographers, are thus central rather than peripheral to competent medical practice.

One emphasis that unites current discussions of ethnographic approaches in anthropology with current discussions of health policy in the UK is a focus on experience. *The Operating Framework for the NHS in England 2010/11* (Department of Health, 2009) identifies the measurement and improvement of patient experience as a national priority. Experience has also become a focus in recent medical anthropology approaches, which attempt to understand the experience of others, often through attempting to approximate their experiences or at least 'walk a mile in their shoes' (Desjarlais, 1992, 1994; Good et al., 1992; Kleinman and Kleinman, 1997; Kleinman, 1999; Wacquant 2004). Approaches to other modes of experience are typically accompanied by continuous reflexive examination and questioning of the ethnographer's own habitual mode of experience. In my own clinical ethnographic research on health issues among Native Americans (Calabrese, 2008, in press), I used interviews and observation but I also learned about practices through doing them and reflecting on the experience, including treating patients at a local Native American clinic, attending a variety of healing ceremonies, and getting to know members of the local community during my two years of fieldwork.

Experientially focused clinical ethnography can provide thickly descriptive, contextualized data on the experiences of patients, carers, and clinicians, transmitting a quasi-experiential understanding to the reader and engaging the reader's imagination and empathy. In opening up to the patient and to the discovery of new information, we go beyond the narrow focus on level of satisfaction to a view of the entire experience of the patient in context. We also go beyond a narrow focus on patients' 'experiences of care' to a holistic understanding of their entire health experience. This includes patients' understandings of their illness and possible treatments, study of the influence of social and cultural contexts, patients' views of medical bureaucracies and policy debates, and the impact of experiential states on the body and health. Research on the quality of care at particular hospitals can enlighten policy

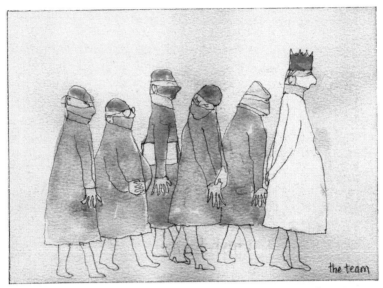

Fig. 3.1 'The Team'. Reproduced with kind permission from Nick Wadley, *Man + Doctor*, Dalkey Archive Press, London, UK, Copyright© 2012 Nick Wadley.

but so can research on the nature of patients' broad experiences of illness and treatment (see Figure 3.1).

Learning about patients' perspectives may help clinicians learn to adjust to these perspectives and more effectively communicate and intervene. Provision of healthcare involves the coming together of the provider's perspective and the patient's perspective and, as I found in my studies of patients' views of treatment at teaching hospitals in the area of Boston, Massachusetts (Calabrese, 2011), patients pay a lot of attention to the quality of their relationship with their provider. However, we must go beyond study of the dynamics of the therapeutic relationship as well. We must see these relationships in the context of society, culture, and policy. Early conceptual models of patient centredness and cultural competence focused on how healthcare providers and patients interact at the interpersonal level. More recent conceptual models have expanded to consider how patients might be treated by the healthcare system as a whole. In fact, even the therapeutic relationship is increasingly shaped and constrained by larger policy structures. For example, increasingly in the USA, interposed between the doctor and patient are new physician incentive systems, impersonal rules that may result in denials of care, and even gag orders through which managed care systems limit the information that doctors can give patients relevant to their treatment. As I found in my Boston study, these changes have undermined patient trust and have caused many patients to view doctors as agents of the state, managed care companies, or drug companies rather than the ally of patients. In short, we need to be patient-centred but we also need to study contextual factors.

Limitations of the method and special responsibilities

The main limitation of ethnographic methods is that they are time consuming. They may require a personal sacrifice on the part of the ethnographer, who may suspend his or her usual living situation and social relations for months or years at a time. There is also the inevitable subjectivity of the ethnographer discussed earlier as well as the potential for bias, given the fact that the ethnographer is dependent upon maintaining positive field relations for research access. In addition, this method is often misunderstood as messy or lacking rigour by those who equate research with highly structured data collection, a high number of participants, and measurement of statistical significance.

There is also a special responsibility that goes along with forming personal relationships with people in the field and collecting their stories, especially with those who are suffering from a particular illness or an adverse socioeconomic situation. As Kleinman and Kleinman (1997) suggest, professional appropriations of suffering have important moral implications: 'To what uses are experiences of suffering put?'. The intimacy of ethnographic research requires careful ethical examination of our interactions with other people and our representations of them.

The ethical imperative of ethnography

I will end with a brief discussion of the ethical rationale for ethnography and health experience research more broadly. The early medical approaches of small-scale societies described by anthropologists utilized less biotechnologically sophisticated methods, but are remarkable to us for the way the entire society gathered around the sick person and sacrificed their time to express their support in healing rituals that could extend for many days.

With the rise of highly technical medical interventions, competence increased but healing became bureaucratized. The embrace of society became a technical and bureaucratic embrace. Dissatisfaction with this impersonal, bureaucratized approach to healing is among the most common findings of health experience research. In my study of patients' experiences of treatment at Boston-area teaching hospitals (Calabrese, 2011), I found that patients tended to describe good medical care as involving an interactive form of communication that blends listening and active problem-solving and in which the patient is viewed 'as a person' rather than as 'a patient'. The most prominent aspects of negative clinical encounters discussed by patients in this study depicted elite clinicians with inflated egos viewing patients as 'specimens' and acting in an authoritarian manner without an obvious concern for the patient. Several patients mentioned that an encounter with such a clinician gave them a negative impression of the entire hospital or caused them to avoid seeking treatment generally.

These findings foreground the continuing importance of the patient's experience of human relationships, meanings, communication, and trust even in an age of sophisticated medical technologies. How can we decrease the patient's feeling of being dehumanized in an impersonal healthcare bureaucracy? The challenge, as I see it, is to keep the high level of technological competence we have developed while we recover what was lost. How can we make healing human again? How can the patient's voice be heard again by the healing system?

In its concern for hearing the patient and taking the patient's experience seriously, clinical ethnography can help us address these challenges. From the perspective of ethics, people who are the objects of medicine should be able to express themselves and their needs. They should have some level of input on a system that has such a significant role in their lives. Their voices should be heard as directly as possible, which means inclusion of narrative data elicited with relatively unstructured interviews and participant observation. We need to hear a plurality of voices and should welcome pluralism in rigorous methodological approaches to research on health experiences.

Further reading

Good, B.J. (1994). *Medicine, rationality and experience: An anthropological perspective.* Cambridge: Cambridge University Press.

Hammersley, M. and Atkinson, P. (1995). *Ethnography: Principles in practice* (2nd edn). London: Routledge.

Helman, C. (2007). *Culture, health and illness.* London: Hodder Arnold.

Kleinman, A. (1988). *The illness narratives: Suffering, healing and the human condition.* New York, NY: Basic Books.

Lambert, H. and McKevitt, C. (2002). Anthropology in health research: from qualitative methods to multidisciplinarity. *British Medical Journal, 325,* 210–13.

References

Biehl, J. (2006). Will to live: AIDS drugs and local economies of salvation. *Public Culture*, *18*(3), 457–72.

Calabrese, J.D. (2008). Clinical paradigm clashes: ethnocentric and political barriers to Native American efforts at self-healing. *Ethos: Journal of the Society for Psychological Anthropology*, *36*(3), 334–53.

Calabrese, J.D. (2011). 'The culture of medicine' as revealed in patients' perspectives on their psychiatric treatment. In: Good, M., *et al.* (eds) *Shattering culture: American medicine responds to cultural diversity*, pp. 184–99. New York, NY: Russell Sage Foundation.

Calabrese, J.D. (in press). *A different medicine: Postcolonial healing in the Native American church*. New York, NY: Oxford University Press.

Caudill, W. (1958). *The psychiatric hospital as a small society*. Cambridge, MA: Harvard University Press.

Department of Health. (2009). *The operating framework for the NHS in England 2010/11*. London: Department of Health.

Desjarlais, R. (1992). Imaginary gardens with real roads. In: Desjarlais, R. (ed.) *Body and emotion*, pp. 3–35. Philadelphia, PA: University of Pennsylvania Press.

Desjarlais, R. (1994). Struggling along: the possibilities for experience among the homeless mentally ill. *American Anthropologist*, *96*(4), 886–901.

Devereux, G. (1961). *Mohave ethnopsychiatry and suicide: The psychiatric knowledge and the psychic disturbances of an Indian tribe*. Washington, DC: Smithsonian.

DiGiacomo, S. (1987). Biomedicine as a cultural system: an anthropologist in the kingdom of the sick. In: Baer, H. (ed.) *Encounters with biomedicine: Case studies in medical anthropology*, pp. 315–46. New York, NY: Gordon and Breach.

Farmer, P. (2004). An anthropology of structural violence. *Current Anthropology*, *45*(3), 305–25.

Garro, L. (1988). Explaining high blood pressure: variation in knowledge about illness. *American Anthropologist*, *15*, 98–119.

Geertz, C. (1973). *The interpretation of cultures*. New York, NY: Basic Books.

Goffman, E. (1961). *Asylums: Essays on the social situation of mental patients and other inmates*. New York, NY: Doubleday.

Good, B.J. (1977). The heart of what's the matter: the semantics of illness in Iran. *Culture, Medicine and Psychiatry*, *1*, 25–58.

Good, B.J. (1994). *Medicine, rationality and experience: An anthropological perspective*. Cambridge: Cambridge University Press.

Good, B.J. and Good, M. (1993). 'Learning medicine': the construction of medical knowledge at Harvard medical school. In: Lindenbaum, S. and Lock, M. (eds). *Knowledge, power, practice*, pp. 81–107. Berkeley, CA: University of California Press.

Good, B.J., *et al.* (1982). Reflexivity and countertransference in a psychiatric cultural consultation clinic. *Culture, Medicine and Psychiatry*, *6*, 281–303.

Good, M., *et al.* (eds) (1992). *Pain as human experience: An anthropological perspective*. Berkeley, CA: University of California Press.

Herdt, G. and Stoller, R. (1990). *Intimate communications: Erotics and the study of culture*. New York, NY: Columbia University Press.

Katz, P. (1981). Ritual in the operating room. *Ethnology*, *20*(4), 335–50.

Kleinman, A. (1980). *Patients and healers in the context of culture*. Berkeley, CA: University of California Press.

Kleinman, A. (1999). Experience and its moral modes: culture, human conditions, and disorder. *Tanner Lectures on Human Values*, *20*, 355–420.

Kleinman, A. and Kleinman, J. (1997). The appeal of experience; the dismay of images: cultural appropriations of suffering in our times. In Kleinman, A., Das, V., and Lock, M. (eds) *Social suffering*, pp. 1–24. Berkeley, CA: University of California Press.

Kleinman, A., Das, V., and Lock, M. (eds) (1997). *Social suffering*. Berkeley, CA: University of California Press.

Koehn, P. (2006). Globalization, migration health, and educational preparation for transnational medical encounters. *Globalization and Health*, 2006, *2*, 2. Available at <http://www.globalizationandhealth.com/content/2/1/2>.

Littlewood, R. and Lipsedge, M. (1982). *Aliens and alienists: Ethnic minorities and psychiatry*. Harmondsworth: Penguin Books.

Luhrmann, T. (2000). *Of two minds: The growing disorder in American psychiatry*. New York, NY: Alfred A. Knopf.

Malinowski, B. (1922). *Argonauts of the Western Pacific*. London: Routledge.

Mattingly, C. (1994). The concept of therapeutic 'emplotment'. *Social Science and Medicine*, *38*, 811–22.

Mead, M. (1928). *Coming of age in Samoa*. New York, NY: William Morrow.

Rubinstein, R. and Lane, S. (1990). International health and development. In Johnson, T. and Sargent, C. (eds) *Medical anthropology: A handbook of theory and method*, pp. 367–90. New York, NY: Praeger.

Sanjek, R. (1990). *Fieldnotes: The makings of anthropology*. Ithaca, NY: Cornell University Press.

Wacquant, L. (2004). *Body & soul: Notebooks of an apprentice boxer*. New York, NY: Oxford University Press.

Whyte, W. (1993). *Street-corner society: The social structure of an Italian slum* (4th edn). Chicago, IL: University of Chicago Press. (Original work published 1943.)

Chapter 4

Observing interactions as an approach to understanding patients' experiences

Fiona Stevenson

This chapter examines observations of interactions as a method for understanding people's experiences of healthcare. Focusing on naturally occurring interactions, it considers how patients' experiences may be understood through observations of the 'work' carried out in consultations. It outlines how observational research is conducted and different approaches to data analysis. Finally it assesses the strengths and limitations of observational research and its use in conjunction with other research approaches.

Using observations to understand health experiences

Interactions between medical staff and patients lie at the heart of the delivery of health services and are important in determining the success of medical outcomes. Detailed analysis of interactional data helps us to understand how the 'work' of consultations is achieved. Observations of interactions elucidate communication in relation to particular medical goals. Relevant work includes the identification of medical agendas (Barry et al., 2000, Heritage et al., 2006), prescribing (Stivers, 2007), and optimizing communication. Drew et al. (2001) used conversation analytic work to show how what doctors choose to say has consequences for what patients go on to say and do and hence for patient participation. This is in keeping with Heritage et al.'s (2006) intervention to examine the effect of the format of questions designed to elicit patients' concerns in consultations: family practitioners used one of two different question formats to elicit additional issues the patient might want to raise. A question using the word 'some' ('Is there *some*thing else you want to address in the visit today?') was compared to one using the word 'any' ('Is there *any*thing else you want to address in the visit today?'). Framing inquiries using 'some' (which has positive polarity) elicited significantly more concerns than 'any' (which has negative polarity). Observational work has also been used to identify barriers and opportunities to more equal participation, shared decision-making, and shared understanding (Ariss, 2009). This work has implications for practice and medical education.

Observational work addressing policy goals has demonstrated potential problems associated with 'one size fits all' pronouncements. Roberts et al.'s (2005) work on misunderstandings demonstrated that although the policy focus is often on people who do not speak English, it is equally if not more important to consider the effect of the ways in which English is spoken by people with limited English, or people who speak variants of English. This work led to the development of a video for general practitioners that can be used in medical education. Trigger material drawn from the research data provides examples of how misunderstandings can be prevented and repaired. Similarly, the complexities involved in how and when interpreters are used may be understood from observational work (Watermeyer, 2011). Findings such as these can help inform the development of acceptable, patient-centred policies.

Observational research elucidates issues that are known to be problematic. Bailey (2008) examined the ways in which people present themselves and their symptoms so as to demonstrate the 'doctorability' of their symptoms and legitimize claims for medical attention. Her research focused on coughs and colds which are at risk of a 'no problem' diagnosis. She demonstrated how coughing in particular places in the consultation resulted in changes in the trajectory of talk between doctors and patients and facilitated resistance by patients of a 'no problem' diagnosis.

Interactions in medical consultations are subject to the same constraints evident in everyday conversation. In English, direct disagreement is interactionally 'dispreferred' (Pomerantz, 1984), meaning people generally work to avoid it. Stivers (2007) examined the ways in which lobbying for antibiotic treatment was constructed by patients and managed by doctors; she demonstrates how doctors use interactional resources to avoid medically inappropriate prescribing.

Video recording allows for deeper understandings by exploring gesture and bodily conduct in interactions. Heath (2002) examined the ways in which gesture and other forms of bodily conduct are used to transform symptoms into suffering as patients 'display, enact and (re)embody medical problems and difficulties', supplementing and supporting their verbal explanations in an active attempt to reveal their experiences of illness. Heath (1984) also presents a detailed account of patients' use of gaze to maintain a state of mutual involvement and sustain integration (see Figure 4.1).

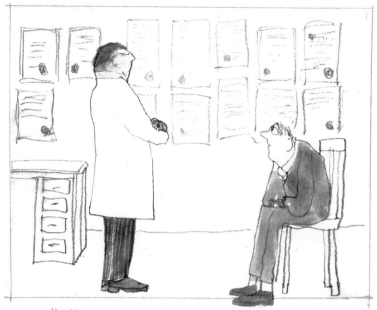

consultation

Fig. 4.1 'Consultation'. Reproduced with kind permission from Nick Wadley, *Man + Doctor*, Dalkey Archive Press, London, UK, Copyright© 2012 Nick Wadley.

Observational work is also useful when considering other forms of non-vocal interaction. Watermeyer and Penn (2009) examined the use of visual props, such as medicine containers, to supplement pharmacists' explanations of dosage instructions and assist with verifying patients' understanding of instructions where pharmacists and patients did not share a common language.

It is important to note that health experiences have been considered using observations in a number of different settings including telemedicine (Pappas and Seale, 2009), primary care (Heritage and Maynard, 2006), pharmacy (Watermeyer and Penn, 2009; Watermeyer, 2011), nurse–patient interaction (Collins, 2005), and health visitor–client interaction (Heritage and Sefi, 1992). This enables reflection on patients' experiences and how interaction is achieved and maintained in various settings with their associated structural constraints.

Conducting observation research

A key task when conducting observation research is gaining access to the research setting. The choice of setting is generally dictated by the area of interest and access is then negotiated, but research opportunities and associated access may also be opportunistic. Thus Silverman (1987) described how a chance meeting gave him access to paediatric congenital heart disease clinics.

The role of the researcher in observational research is important; in particular, their personal characteristics, which will affect the way in which people interact with them. The researcher generally has to work to gain acceptance in the research setting, particularly with people who are more junior than the person who officially granted access, but at the same time avoid becoming so immersed that they no longer notice what is different or interesting about the setting (see Chapter 3).

The particular ethical and governance permissions required in health settings may prove challenging and affect the research design and what it is possible to observe. In addition to formal requirements, decisions have to be made about how to explain studies so that they are ethically robust and people are able to make an informed decision about participation, yet do not start altering their behaviour in response to being informed of specific areas of interest.

The research setting dictates, to a great extent, the possibilities for observation. For example, clinics are semi-public spaces in which it may be possible to unobtrusively observe behaviours, make notes, and even record interactions. Silverman (1987), in his study of hospital clinics, used observational notes and a tape recorder and discussed how this was possible as people were used to notes being taken and a tape recorder could easily be set up in advance.

Recording is better suited to focused, bounded situations such as a consultation than a less structured, semi-informal setting like a waiting room, where it may be more appropriate to take notes of observations of interest. In such situations checklists may prove useful. A good memory for detail is an asset, coupled with as much note taking as appears feasible in the setting without causing disruption. Audio or video recording of consultations may minimize disruption on the research setting from the researcher, but replaces it with the potentially disruptive effect of the recording equipment and its operation. Recording interactions does overcome the problem of recall and selectivity of note taking; however, it does not diminish the need for decisions about what is observed and what is subsequently transcribed and analysed.

When recording interactions, there is a strong preference for video over audio recording. Video is judged to provide access to the complex forms of social interaction and collaboration that underpin healthcare (Heath et al., 2007). Yet there are problems associated with the acceptability and practicality of video as opposed to audio recordings. Heritage and Sefi (1992), in their study of interactions between health visitors and first-time mothers, selected audio recording as a straightforward technique for data collection that could be used by the health visitors themselves. They felt the process of video recording would have constituted an intrusive distraction in a delicate setting. (For more discussion of this see Chapter 7 on story-gathering and Chapter 5 on narrative interviewing.) They however also discussed the drawbacks of using audio as opposed to video recordings, notably the impossibility of determining the spatial arrangement of the parties to the interaction and, on many occasions, the possibly important non-vocal activities of the parties. They acknowledged this limited the possibilities for analysis and consequently the conclusions that can be drawn.

Analysis of observational data

Observations are analysed in a number of ways. Decisions about analysis may be based on the epistemological position of the researcher but may also reflect practical issues such as the resources available. Analysis decisions determine transcription decisions. The least resource-intensive approach may mean data are not transcribed; rather analysis is based on field notes in combination with listening/viewing recordings. A similar approach may be to only transcribe key sections. Where coding frameworks or thematic analysis are used then generally a word-for-word transcription will be conducted, often by a trained transcriber rather than the researcher. At the extreme are methods such as conversation analysis (CA) which requires detailed, fine-grained transcription, noting features such as pauses, in and out breaths, hesitations, and overlaps. Initially a word-for-word transcription may be produced and this will be used alongside the video/audio recording in order to identify aspects of interest which may then be transcribed in more detail. The detailed and labour intensive transcription work will typically be carried out by the researcher.

CA is commonly used to analyse observational data. CA is characterized by fine-grained analysis examining the 'work' done in interactions and the production of social actions. The focus remains at all times on what is directly observable in the data and the effect on interactional uptake by other participants. A key tenet is that analysis should not be constrained by the wider context in which interactions take place or prior theoretical assumptions; therefore pre-existing categorizations such as gender and age are not employed as part of the analysis. It is argued that if these differences are important they will become apparent in detailed analysis so there is no need to impose constructions such as these on the data. Such characterizations may, however, be used to introduce an extract once analysis is complete and the data are presented for publication.

Drew et al. (2001) argued that CA offers a rigorous method which is applicable to large data sets. A fundamental tenet of CA is that interaction is a collaborative process. Thus CA involves detailed sequential analysis to explore how speakers design the content of each of their 'turns' at talking and to look at how interactions are sequenced and managed. Any utterances and indeed many aspects of non-verbal behaviour are considered to be performing social actions of various kinds. Utterances and actions are seen as connected in sequences of actions, so that what one participant says and does is generated by, and dependent upon, what the other has said and done. The identification of sequential patterns, and the practices through which these patterns are generated, are distinctive to CA's approach. Once a practice is identified, large-scale data corpora are examined to collect as many examples as possible of that practice.

Discourse analysis (DA) often adopts a similar detailed micro-level approach to the analysis of observation data but differs from CA as it examines features outside of the directly observable properties of data, such as speakers' background and audience, their choice of vocabulary, grammar, intonation, and the use of rhetoric which is considered to be part of the wider context within which talk occurs. Yet in practice, divisions between analyses are not necessarily clear cut, for example, Watermeyer and Penn (2009) used a hybrid approach incorporating aspects of CA and theme-orientated DA in their study of the use of props to facilitate communication in multilingual pharmacy interactions.

Coding frameworks are commonly used in observation research in order to categorize and assess communication in relation to particular aspects of interest. There are well-known frameworks such as the Roter interaction analysis system (RIAS) (Roter and Larson, 2002), which is designed to implement an exhaustive classification of the events of the medical visit. Coding frameworks are also developed for particular purposes, for example, delineating the intricacies of physician–patient discussions to better understand the range of communication about new prescriptions (Tarn et al., 2008). Observational data may also be subject to thematic analysis, for example, Britten et al. (2000) used thematic analysis of consultation data to consider misunderstandings in primary care consultations.

The same data may be analysed in different ways in order to answer different research questions. Thus data thematically analysed to support Britten et al.'s (2000) work on misunderstandings in primary care consultations was reanalysed using CA to consider patient participation in relation to the elicitation of the initial concern in opening sequences of primary care consultations and the formulation of patients' problems (Gafaranga and Britten, 2007).

Finally, decisions about analysis may be at least partially determined by external factors. Silverman (1987) explains that he had insufficient time to prepare the precise transcripts used in CA in order to analyse observations from clinics. The workload implications would have meant only a tiny proportion of the tapes could have been used. He chose instead to apply an existing theoretical framework to his data, namely 'a Goffman-based model of the "ceremonial order" of the clinic'.

Strengths and limitations of observational research

Observational work provides an understanding of what is happening in a naturalist setting considering issues which are so embedded in everyday interactions that they are impossible to investigate using any other method. It considers the whole research setting and both processes and interactions may be observed. Crucially data are not a response to particular questions or prompts from the researcher; rather observational methods focus on what people do rather than what they say they do (see Chapter 3).

Observational research is, however, resource intensive in relation to skills and requires an academic apprenticeship and dedicated supervision. Fieldwork and analysis are very labour intensive and there is little opportunity for reducing the burden through division of labour. Practically, negotiating access and acceptance in a research setting may prove problematic, while the presence of a researcher and/or recording equipment may affect interactions.

Observations in conjunction with other research approaches

Observations are often carried out in tandem with methods such as interviewing and questionnaires enabling interactional data to be considered alongside accounts of actions. As an example, a study of doctor–patient communication about medicines combined (1) interviews conducted with patients before and after their consultation in general practice, (2) interviews with doctors following the consultation, and (3) audio-taped recordings of the consultation. Data were combined to present insights on a range of patients' experiences such as the extent of shared decision-making in doctor–patient communication about drugs (Stevenson et al., 2000), expressions of the lifeworld in consultations (Barry et al., 2001), misunderstandings in general practice prescribing decisions (Britten et al., 2000), the expression of aversion to medicines in general practice consultations (Britten et al., 2004), self-treatment and its discussion in medical consultations (Stevenson et al., 2003), the influence of perceptions of legitimacy on medicine-taking and prescribing (Stevenson et al., 2002), and patients' unvoiced agendas in general practice consultations (Barry et al., 2000). Follow-up work was conducted using a similar design, but including a questionnaire before and after the consultation and telephone (rather than face-to-face) interviews to examine adherence. The aim was to test the robustness as a research design for clinicians to then use to assess their own practice (Jenkins et al., 2003). All this work fed into the development of the 'concordance' model of communication between healthcare professionals and patients (Bond, 2004). A key focus of this work was translating conceptual work around concordance into undergraduate and postgraduate medical education and encouraging the incorporation of the ideas into health policy and guidelines for practice.

While combining data collected using different research methods may be fruitful, it may prove difficult for researchers to manage and interpret data collected using different approaches, which in practice rarely triangulate around a common story. Silverman (1987) obtained funding to conduct a study of interactions in hospital clinics which included observations and interviews. Although combining observational and interview data is well accepted, he reported struggling to find a suitable framework and a methodology for analysing the interview data and combining it with the observational data.

Discussion

Observations of interactions in healthcare elucidate our understanding of people's health experiences. Understandings can be developed from the perspective of an outside observer which differs from, though may be complemented by, the perspective obtained by asking people for their views and opinions. Observations are particularly useful for identifying problems in interaction, understanding how problems may occur, and when they do occur, how they are addressed. Certain interactional problems may be specific to medical consultations or may reflect more general problems also experienced outside of medical consultations.

A particular strength of observational research is the ability to consider the role and importance of non-vocal interaction such as gesture. Such research requires video data. Decisions made in relation to data collection and analysis crucially affect the scope of what can ultimately be known. Such decisions are affected by practical considerations, such as the acceptability and practicality of using video as opposed to audio recording for data collection. Similarly, decisions about analysis may also be affected by practical considerations, such as the time available.

Health policy in many countries (see Chapter 15) is supporting greater patient involvement in healthcare decisions. In this climate, observational work and associated detailed analysis can be used to identify potential problem areas in relation to current health policy and opportunities for approaches such as patient-centred care, shared decision-making, and the use of patient reported outcome measures or survey evidence in management (see Chapters 8 and 9). It may also inform medical education, supplementing and complementing existing teaching about patient-centred care.

Finally, it is important to recognize that when examining health experiences, observations may complement, and be complemented by, the use of other methods of data collection such as interviews, focus groups, and questionnaires.

Conclusions

The key strength of observational research is the opportunity to explore processes and interactions from the perspective of an outsider, free from researchers' prompts. Crucially, observational research shines a light on issues which are 'normalized' and so embedded in the everyday interactions and social structures of healthcare that they are impossible to investigate using any other approach.

Further reading

Bailey, J. (2008). Could patients' coughing have communicative significance? *Communication & Medicine*, 5, 105–15.

Heath, C. (2002). Demonstrative suffering: the gestural (re) embodiment of symptoms. *Journal of Communication*, 52, 597–616.

Roberts, C., *et al*. (2005). Misunderstandings: a qualitative study of primary care consultations in multilingual settings, and educational implications. *Medical Education*, 39, 465–75.

Silverman, D. (1987). *Communication in medical practice. Social relations in the clinic*. London: Sage.

Watermeyer, J. (2011). 'She will hear me': how a flexible interpreting style enables patients to manage the inclusion of interpreters in mediated pharmacy interactions. *Health Communication*, 26, 71–81.

References

Ariss, S.M. (2009). Asymmetrical knowledge claims in general practice consultations with frequently attending patients: limitations and opportunities for patient participation. *Social Science and Medicine*, 69, 908–19.

Bailey, J. (2008). Could patients' coughing have communicative significance? *Communication & Medicine*, 5, 105–15.

Barry, C.A., *et al.* (2000). Patients' unvoiced agendas in general practice consultations. *British Medical Journal, 320*, 1246–50.

Barry, C.A., *et al.* (2001). Giving voice to the lifeworld. More humane, more effective medical care? *Social Science & Medicine, 53*, 487–505.

Bond, C. (ed.) (2004). *Concordance*. London: Pharmaceutical Press.

Britten, N., *et al.* (2000). Misunderstandings in general practice prescribing decisions: a qualitative study. *British Medical Journal. 320*, 484–8.

Britten, N., *et al.* (2004). The expression of aversion to medicines in general practice consultations. *Social Science and Medicine, 59*, 1495–503.

Collins, S. (2005). Explanations in consultations: the combined effectiveness of doctors' and nurses' communication with patients. *Medical Education, 39*, 785–96.

Drew, P., Chatwin, J., and Collins, S. (2001). Conversation analysis: a method for research into interactions between patients and health-care professionals. *Health Expectations, 4*, 58–70.

Gafaranga, J. and Britten, N. (2007). Patient participation in formulating and opening sequences. In: Collins, S., *et al.* (eds.) *Patient participation in health care consultations. Qualitative perspectives*, pp. 104–20. Maidenhead: Open University Press.

Heath, C. (1984). Participation in the medical consultation: the co-ordination of verbal and nonverbal behaviour between the doctor and the patient. *Sociology of Health and Illness, 6*, 311–38.

Heath, C. (2002). Demonstrative suffering: the gestural (re) embodiment of symptoms. *Journal of Communication, 52*, 597–616.

Heath, C., Luff, P., and Sanchez Svensson, M. (2007). Video and qualitative research: analysing medical practice and interaction. *Medical Education, 41*, 109–16.

Heritage, J. and Sefi, S. (1992). Dilemmas of advice: aspects of the delivery and reception of advice in interactions between health visitors and first time mothers. In: Drew, P. and Heritage, J. (eds) *Talk at work*, pp. 359–417. Cambridge: Cambridge University Press.

Heritage, J, *et al.* (2006). Reducing patients' unmet concerns in primary care: the difference one word can make. *Journal of General Internal Medicine, 22*, 1429–33.

Heritage, J. and Maynard, D.W. (eds) (2006). *Communication in medical care. Interaction between primary care physicians and patients*. Cambridge: Cambridge University Press.

Jenkins, L., *et al.* (2003). Developing and using qualitative instruments for measuring doctor-patient communication about drugs. *Patient Education and Counseling, 50*, 273–8.

Pappas, Y. and Seale, C. (2009). The opening phase of telemedicine consultations: an analysis of interaction. *Social Science & Medicine, 68*, 1229–37.

Pomerantz, A. (1984). Agreeing and disagreeing with assessments: some features of preferred/dispreferred turn shapes. In: Atkinson, J.M. and Heritage, J. (eds) *Structures of social action. Studies in conversation analysis*, pp. 57–101. Cambridge: Cambridge University Press.

Roberts, C., *et al.* (2005). Misunderstandings: a qualitative study of primary care consultations in multilingual settings, and educational implications. *Medical Education, 39*, 465–75.

Roter, D. and Larson, S. (2002). The Roter interaction analysis system (RIAS): utility and flexibility for analysis of medical interactions. *Patient Education and Counseling, 46*, 243–51.

Silverman, D. (1987). *Communication in medical practice. Social relations in the clinic.* London: Sage.

Stevenson, F.A., *et al.* (2000) Doctor—patient communication about drugs: the evidence for shared decision making. *Social Science and Medicine, 50,* 829–40.

Stevenson, F.A., *et al.* (2002). Perceptions of legitimacy: the influence on medicine-taking and prescribing. *Health, 6,* 85–104.

Stevenson, F.A., *et al.* (2003). Self treatment and its discussion in medical consultations: how is medical pluralism managed in practice? *Social Science and Medicine, 57,* 513–27.

Stivers, T. (2007). *Prescribing under pressure. Parent-physician conversations and antibiotics.* New York, NY: Oxford University Press.

Tarn, D.M., *et al.* (2008). Prescribing new medications: a taxonomy of physician-patient communication. *Communication & Medicine, 5,* 195–208.

Watermeyer, J. and Penn, C. (2009). 'Come let me show you': the use of props to facilitate communication of antiviral dosage instructions in multilingual pharmacy interactions. In: Lagerwerf, L., Boer, H., and Wasserman, H. (eds) *Health communication in Southern Africa: Engaging with social and cultural diversity,* pp. 191–216. Amsterdam: Rozenberg publishers.

Watermeyer, J. (2011). 'She will hear me': how a flexible interpreting style enables patients to manage the inclusion of interpreters in mediated pharmacy interactions. *Health Communication, 26,* 71–81.

Chapter 5

Narrative interviewing

Sue Ziebland

Introduction

People bleed stories. Academics gather narratives.

Reproduced from Unni Wikan,
With life in one's lap: the story of an eye/i (or two).
In: Cheryl Mattingly and Linda Garro (eds)
Narrative and the cultural construction of illness and healing,
p. 217, University of California Press, Berkeley, Copyright © 2000.

Narrative interviewing is a method of collecting people's accounts, or stories, of their experiences. The method can be applied to many different areas of life and draws on approaches commonly used in oral history, anthropology, and sociology. Narrative interviews, in common with other qualitative methods, tend to address 'how' and 'why' questions rather than 'how many' or cause and effect questions.

The approach is mostly valued as a style of interview that seeks to get close to what is most important to respondents (who in healthcare might be patients, family carers, health professionals, or members of the public) through encouraging an account of their own perspectives and priorities, using the terms and language that they prefer. The method is used widely in social science-informed health research literature to address broad research questions such as 'What are the experiences of people who are diagnosed with lung cancer?', rather than more focused questions like 'What are the financial support needs of people diagnosed with lung cancer?', that might use a more structured interview method. A research design might combine narrative and semi-structured interview techniques, or employ unstructured interviews with ethnographic observations (Chapter 3) or survey methods (Chapter 9).

The growth of narrative research

Several authors have referred (approvingly or otherwise) to an 'exponential' growth in narrative research since the 1980s. To add some numbers to this impression, and to examine which areas of scholarship have embraced narratives most enthusiastically, we searched the literature (in February 2012) on the 'Web of Science' database which covers sciences, social sciences, arts, and humanities. The search included narrative (with 'interviewing' or 'interviews' or 'inquiry'); yielding 646 results, which were plotted against the year when they were published. Figure 5.1 demonstrates the slow increase in the 1990s and marked upward trend since the turn of the century. Narrative approaches are particularly prominent in social science studies in health journals (58% of the papers in our literature search were in this category) and in education journals (26%).

This chapter considers the application of an interview method from qualitative social science which is used to gather and analyse health narratives; the findings are sometimes (but not always) intended to inform clinical practice or the delivery or organization of health services. A parallel and distinct development, which draws on some of the same ideas as narrative research, concerns the therapeutic potential both of storytelling for patients (Pennebaker, 2000) and of story listening by health professionals. Sometimes called 'narrative-based medicine' this approach encourages clinicians to elicit patients' narratives in the clinical context (listen to the patient's story...) to improve diagnostics and treatment and benefit the therapeutic alliance between patient and professional. Family doctors, general practitioners, psychiatrists, and

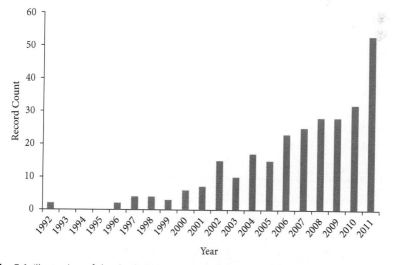

Fig. 5.1 Illustration of the rise in 'narrative' research in health-related articles 1996–2011. Data derived from Web of Science® prepared by THOMSON REUTERS®, Inc. (Thomson®), Philadelphia, Pennsylvania, USA.

other health professionals (Hurwitz et al., 2004) have argued that listening to the patient's story is not only respectful and humane but can also be more efficient than a purely medical model, which a body of research has demonstrated can result in misunderstandings and inefficiencies in care (Chapter 4).

Conducting narrative interviews

Narrative interviews differ from more structured interview methods in several ways. Bauer (1996) describes three ways that a structured interview imposes the research agenda: in the selection of the themes and topics, the ordering of the questions, and the wording of the questions. In contrast, a narrative interview is intended to gather the respondent's own perspectives. Lack of focus may be a criticism in some contexts, but in the narrative interview it can mean that the respondent's perspective is not constrained by the researcher's agenda.

This does not mean that the researcher necessarily enters the interview in a state of naïvety about the health condition; even if they did, this naïvety would inevitably be compromised after the first few interviews. Rather, the interviewer offers the participant the opportunity to control the direction and content of the interview. Similarly, the *participant* will not be able to make an informed decision to agree to an interview unless they are given at least some inkling of what the topic might be. Before the interview begins the researcher is likely to explain what she or he is interested in hearing about, although this might be presented in very general terms such as 'living with chronic illness'.

The direction of the conversation and the topics discussed are thus largely in the hands of the participant, who decides what they want to say, how to structure their account, and, of course, what not to say. In narrative interviewing the interviewee may be positioned as a 'storyteller' rather than a 'respondent'.

A narrative interview would typically start with an open-ended question, intended to elicit the person's accounts of their experience. While it is unlikely that a request for an 'illness narrative' would be very fruitful in the context of most interviews, one might ask a question such as 'Could you tell me about what's happened since you first suspected a problem?'. Even when the narrator has no idea where the story will end, the beginning may be identifiable. For example, anthropologist Unni Wikan, in her account of the aftermath of a detached retina, explains that she can identify the beginning of her story because 'the beginning is the turning point—the end is simply what then happened or how it all went. Life goes on, and so I do not know how it all went; the ending is not yet clear' (Wikan, 2000, p. 215).

Narrative research interviewing skills include establishing rapport and trust, listening attentively to what the participant says, avoiding interruptions, and making a (mental) note of any issues that need to be followed up after the account is complete.

The length of the interview is hard to predict—it could be over in half an hour if the participant has very little to say, or last for several hours, perhaps over a number of sessions if the account is complicated, or the participant is not well enough for a lengthy, one-off interview. For example, among the 3,000 interviews collected in the Health Experiences Research Group (HERG) in Oxford there are a few that last over five hours and others that were complete in around thirty minutes. From an organizational point of view this unpredictability means that it would not normally be advisable to arrange more than one interview in a normal working day.

Ethical issues

Narrative interviewing raises some particular ethical issues since it is not possible to fully inform the participant about the likely content of the interview in advance. While the interview may be seen as more in the participant's control than in most other research approaches, neither the participant nor researcher knows precisely what will be discussed before the interview begins. For this reason, narrative researchers sometimes offer the participant a copy of their interview transcript to review, with the option of removing sections, before a final consent form is signed. Interviews that are collected in HERG for <http://www.healthtalkonline.org> use a two-stage consent and copyright process to ensure that participants are comfortable for extracts from their interview to be used on a website. Approximately 10% of these interviews have some section(s) removed between the interview and copyright stage.

Combining narrative and other interview methods

In health research, narrative methods are often combined with a semi-structured interview. This is particularly useful where the research is designed to explore a relatively wide range of perspectives. Particular topics might be anticipated at the beginning of the study, perhaps through literature review, or they might emerge during early interviews. The researcher may be interested to know if the issue is introduced in a narrative section, but use some follow-up questions if it does not arise unprompted. Whether the issue was raised by the participant in the narrative section, or only in response to specific questioning, is likely to be relevant to the analysis. It is usually preferable to start with the narrative section, then ask supplementary questions (e.g. Can you tell me more about that? What was that experience like for you?) when the account comes to a natural end. If desired, more focused prompts and questions, or even a structured and standardized survey instrument could be used at the end. In this way the narrative section is not unduly influenced by the issues that are raised in the more structured section. If the interview starts with a series of specific items, whether about coping, finances, communication with doctors, treatment decisions, or sex and relationships, it can be difficult, both for the participant and researcher, to realign their focus to the participant's own priorities and perspectives.

Narratives can also be sought within interviews that use a mainly structured approach. For example, a predominately structured (or semi-structured) interview method might include an invitation to narrate a specific example, e.g. 'Could you tell me about a recent occasion when that happened?'. This can shift an account from the general to the specific and gather examples that help the researcher to understand the respondents' perspectives. Switching between structured and unstructured methods in an interview requires flexible research skills or the participant may be unsure what is expected—and the interview may be in danger of breaking down in the confusion.

Analysing narrative interviews

Catherine Riessman reminds us that 'Storytelling, to put the argument simply, is what we do with our research materials and what informants do with us' (Riessman, 1993, p. 1). The analytic task, whichever analytic approach is used, can be seen as identifying a 'story' across the data set. This might be achieved through focusing on the events that are narrated, or on how the narrative itself is structured, or on the meanings the narrator ascribes to the events. Rather than simply relating what people have told us, analysis aims to provide an informed interpretation of their accounts. Some critics (see 'Narrative interviews: concerns and cautions' section) have drawn attention to the lack of theoretically informed analyses in many narrative interview studies. While it is analytically insufficient simply to let interview extracts speak for themselves, the challenge for the analyst is to present enough of the data that the line of argument and interpretation are convincing, while situating the findings in the appropriate theoretical and research literature.

Narrative interviews are usually audio (or video) recorded and transcribed verbatim, with pauses timed and repetitions included. Verbatim transcriptions often highlight the untidiness of speech; even the highly articulate can appear stilted when all pauses, ums, ers, and repetitions are marked. Accurate transcription is important, but the level of detail will vary depending on the type of analysis; a thematic analysis may require standard orthographic transcription while minute attention to detail is required for conversation analysis (Chapter 4). Transcription should be seen as a research act, even if performed by an audio-typist rather than a researcher.

Narrative analysis rarely uses frequency counts, or numerical comparisons, although in some circumstances these can indicate broad patterns in the data. Seale, for example, has used the quantitative technique of comparative keyword analysis to identify differences in language patterns (Seale et al., 2006).

Qualitative approaches to narrative analysis usually attend to how the account is structured as well as what people say (Riessman 1993). However, there is no single approach to analysing narratives; different disciplines have developed a variety of models which reflect their analytic interests. A socio-linguist might use Labov's (1972) model which identifies narrative components as the abstract, orientation, complicating action, evaluation, result or resolution, and possibly a coda. While socio-linguists primarily concern themselves with stories that arise spontaneously in everyday interactions (Thornborrow and Coates, 2005, p. 2) Labov's model can also be used to analyse storytelling in interviews. For example, a story about someone else may be included as a subnarrative. The narrative analyst might consider why this account was told, in this way, at this point in the interview. Cheshire and Ziebland comment on a narrative related by Rose, who was interviewed about her hypertension. She refers to a neighbour who has admitted, in conversation, that she sometimes forgets to take her medicine. In the interview this subnarrative is apparently offered as a point of comparison with Rose's own careful system for remembering to take her medicines (Cheshire and Ziebland, 2005). Narrative interviews can also be analysed as performances of, for example, gender, expertise, or moral identity.

A recent (2012) special issue of the journal *Chronic Illness* demonstrates the very different analytic approaches that can be applied to narrative interviews. Six papers, focused on emotional responses to chronic illness, were all based on narrative interview studies conducted in the UK, Germany, Israel, and Japan. Analytic approaches ranged from a socio-linguistic analysis of how patients positioned their doctors' voices in 394 narrated scenes, extracted from 56 diabetes and chronic pain interviews (Lucius-Hoene et al., 2012) to an interpretative phenomenological analysis of six interviews with Israelis living with chronic pain (Lavie-Ajayi et al., 2012). Locock and colleagues explored how metaphoric language is employed to convey emotions in 46 interviews with people affected by motor neurone disease (Locock et al., 2012). Three of the papers used qualitative thematic analyses to look at *how* people talk as well as *what* they said in (1) accounts of fear in narrative interviews with young British people with epilepsy (Ryan and Räisänen, 2012), (2) frustration in chronic pain (Dow et al., 2012), and (3) communication of cancer prognosis in Japan (Sato et al., 2012). Thus, even though the interview method was very similar, the approaches to analysis differed considerably.

Researchers may decide to check their interpretation of the narrative with their participants. Borland, an American oral historian, tells a cautionary tale about her use of a feminist perspective to interpret an incident from her grandmother's life history. When invited to comment, her grandmother rejected the analysis and argued a different interpretation (Borland, 2006). Borland reflects that while an analysis should stand up to scrutiny, and hopefully one that participants would recognize as a reasonable and respectful interpretation of their account, the value of a scholarly work does not ultimately rest on their approval. Consider, for example, whether one would willingly revise an analysis of interviews with powerful respondents such as politicians or business and media leaders.

Some authors suggest that there may be intrinsic benefits to the participant who is able to narrate the story of their illness. Research in this field has mainly concerned written, rather than oral, narratives but there is some evidence that storytelling may be therapeutic (Pennebaker 2000).

Applications of narrative interviews

Narrative interview collections may either be conducted as stand-alone studies, perhaps to illuminate patients' perspective of illness or the delivery of healthcare, or be used as preliminary study. Unstructured, narrative interviews can sometimes uncover previously unrecognized experiences of clinical care pathways that can then be explored further in qualitative or quantitative studies with a tighter research focus (Chapters 8 and 9). Analysis of narrative interviews may suggest hypotheses to test in quantitative research, identify appropriate outcome variables for assessing the effects of interventions, or inform interview or questionnaire design by clarifying the language and terms commonly used by the respondents. Secondary analysis of existing narrative interviews, collected for another purpose, may provide a cost-effective alternative to new interviews (Heaton, 2004).

Narrative interviews can also provide raw material for resources to encourage service development, or professional training. The website <http://www.patientstories.org> includes powerful films based on interviews about patients' experiences; these are intended to stimulate healthcare providers to improve patient safety. The patients' experiences site <http://www.healthtalkonline.org> features audio and video clips from narrative interviews, presented with analyses from around 40 interviews for each of the many different health conditions covered. Primarily developed as a resource for direct public and patient access, this material is also used in training health and social care professionals, informing National Institute for Health and Clinical Excellence clinical guidelines, and has been re-analysed to provide trigger films for organizational development (see Chapter 14).

Narrative researchers may prefer to publish in specialist journals, rather than clinical and health policy journals, where word lengths tend to be shorter and conclusions may seem too abrupt. This may have reduced the influence of narrative studies on clinical practice in the past. However, the growing emphasis on qualitative literature synthesis (Chapter 11) means that even if the results are originally published for a specialist audience the findings may inform practice in combination with other published research.

Limitations of a narrative approach

While narrative interviewing allows the respondent to control the interview and narrate their story in the way they prefer, it is clear that not everyone relishes participating in this sort of interview. An approach which invites the respondent to tell a story in their own words may be unfamiliar, even challenging, to the participant (Chapter 13). Those who have experience of more structured research, or were expecting the question and answer format of the TV or radio interview, may be flummoxed by an invitation to 'tell a story', even if delivered by an attentive and encouraging qualitative social scientist.

Another limitation relates to scope and generalizability. Narrative researchers may collect only a few interviews and make no particular claims for the reach of their findings. Even those researchers who aim for a broad and diverse sample, to represent a wide range of experiences, are not seeking samples that will be numerically representative. Narrative interview studies, in common with many other qualitative methods, may therefore give little insight into the distribution or frequency of particular perspectives or characteristics in the population.

Narrative interviews: concerns and cautions

In parallel with the rise in narrative research, a few commentators have warned that the approach has sometimes been used in an uncritical, non-sociological, pseudo therapeutic or simply naïve and romanticized manner. While it is not an intention of this chapter to attempt a full rehearsal of these criticisms and cautions, they are likely to be of interest to narrative researchers.

Atkinson (1997) considered the popularity of narrative data and analysis in sociology as a 'mixed blessing'. He notes that the very notion of the in-depth interview 'often carries with it connotations that the surface of the respondent can be probed, and that the personal, private aspects of 'experience' can be rendered visible through dialogue' (1997, p. 327). Woods (2011) identifies several concerns about the use of narratives in medical humanities, including the question of whether an account is authentic. Other concerns include the lack of cultural, historical, and indeed narrative approaches of interpretation and the (rarely discussed) potential for narratives to be used as objects of power, set against people's interests. An account of an illness experience can be moving and memorable but it can also be inappropriately applied, or misleading.

Strawson argues against the claims that there is anything natural, or beneficial, about perceiving and relating one's life as a story; he proposes instead that a life lived as a series of episodes, with no sense of a narrative thread, has every chance of being both rational and satisfying; any assumption that people should be able to provide narrative accounts is therefore flawed (Strawson, 2004).

Shapiro (2011) acknowledges that 'all stories necessarily contain elements of authenticity and inauthenticity, are always partly trustworthy and partly untrustworthy, to some degree are unavoidably self-representations and performances'. This melding of remembered and improvised details in an account is what Bury has described as 'factions' (Bury, 2001). Critical thinking is therefore important, but Shapiro cautions that we should not cease to engage with narratives in a 'compassionate and humble context'. Mishler recognizes that researchers will be concerned by authenticity but notes:

> My intent is to shift attention away from investigator's 'problems' such as technical issues of reliability and validity, to respondents' problems, specifically their efforts to construct coherent and reasonable worlds of meaning and to make sense of their experiences (Mishler, 1991, p. 118).

Scholars recognize the active process of meaning construction that is inherent in an interview; power relations cannot be overcome simply by giving the respondent the floor. As Abma points out (2002), people who are marginalized and excluded also self-censor for other reasons, such as because they 'fear sanctions and find their experiences too painful to confront'. Western society has tended to accord higher status to abstract theories than to people's accounts of their own embodied experiences yet these accounts can 'counter and interrupt official stories and canonised knowledge' (Abma, 2002, p. 20).

Conclusion

The in-depth, narrative interview has become a mainstay of contemporary, qualitative health research. The emphasis on allowing the participant to control the flow and content of the interview aligns with a patient-centred approach in research and practice. Whether presented singly, or collectively, narratives can also be employed to challenge stereotypes and indifference (Bauman, 1993, p. 155).

Further reading

Atkinson, P. (1997). Narrative turn or blind alley? *Qualitative Health Research*, *7*, 325–44.

Kleinman, A. (1988). *The illness narratives: Suffering, healing, and the human condition*. New York, NY: Basic Books.

Mishler, E.G. (1991). *Research interviewing: Context and narrative*. Cambridge, MA: Harvard University Press.

Riessman, C.K. (1993). *Narrative analysis*. Thousand Oaks, CA: Sage.

Woods, A. (2011). The limits of narrative: provocations for the medical humanities. *Medical Humanities*, *37*, 73–8.

References

Abma, T.A. (2002). Emerging narrative forms of knowledge representation in the health sciences: two texts in a postmodern context. *Qualitative Health Research*, *12*, 5–27.

Atkinson, P. (1997). Narrative turn or blind alley? *Qualitative Health Research*, *7*, 325–44.

Bauer, M. (1996). *The narrative interview: Comments on a technique for qualitative data collection*. London: London School of Economics and Political Science, Methodology Institute.

Bauman, Z. (1993). *Postmodern ethics*. Oxford: Blackwell.

Borland, K. (2006). 'That's not what I said': interpretive conflict in oral narrative research. In: Perks, R. and Thomson, A. (eds) *The oral history reader* (2nd edn). London: Routledge.

Bury, M. (2001). Illness narratives: fact or fiction? *Sociology of Health & Illness*, *23*, 263–85.

Cheshire, J. and Ziebland, S. (2005). Narrative as a resource in accounts of the experience of illness. In: Coates, J. and Thornborrow, J. (eds) *The sociolinguistics of narrative*, pp. 17–40. Amsterdam: John Benjamins.

Dow, C.M., Roche, P.A., and Ziebland, S. (2012). Talk of frustration in the narratives of people with chronic pain. *Chronic Illness*, *8*(3), 176–91.

Heaton, J. (2004). *Reworking qualitative data*. London: Sage.

Hurwitz, B., Greenhalgh, T., and Skultans, V. (eds) (2004). *Narrative research in health and illness*. London: BMJ Books.

Kleinman, A. (1988). *The illness narratives: Suffering, healing, and the human condition*. New York, NY: Basic Books.

Labov, W. (1972). *Language in the inner city*. Philadelphia, PA: University of Pennsylvania Press.

Lavie-Ajayi, M., Almog, N., and Krumer-Nevo, M. (2012). Chronic pain as a narratological distress: a phenomenological study. *Chronic Illness*, *8*(3), 192–200.

Locock, L., Mazanderani, F., and Powell, J. (2012). Metaphoric language and the articulation of emotions by people affected by motor neurone disease. *Chronic Illness*, *8*, 201–13.

Lucius-Hoene, G., *et al.* (2012). Doctors' voices in patients' narratives: coping with emotions in storytelling. *Chronic Illness*, *8*, 163–75.

Mishler, E.G. (1991). *Research interviewing: context and narrative*. Cambridge, MA: Harvard University Press.

Pennebaker, J.W. (2000). Telling stories: the health benefits of narrative. *Literature and Medicine*, *19*, 3–18.

Riessman, C.K. (1993). *Narrative analysis*. Thousand Oaks, CA: Sage.

Ryan, S. and Raisanen, U. (2012). 'The brain is such a delicate thing': an exploration of fear and seizures among young people with epilepsy. *Chronic Illness*, *8*, 214–24.

Sato, R.S., *et al.* (2012). The meaning of life prognosis disclosure for Japanese cancer patients: a qualitative study of patients' narratives. *Chronic Illness*, *8*, 225–36.

Seale, C., Charteris-Black, J., and Ziebland, S. (2006). Gender, cancer experience and internet use: a comparative keyword analysis of interviews and online cancer support groups. *Social Science & Medicine*, *62*(10), 2577–90.

Shapiro, J. (2011). Illness narratives: reliability, authenticity and the empathic witness *Medical Humanities*, *37*(2), 68–72.

Strawson, G. (2004). Against narrativity. *Ratio*, *17*, 428–52.

Thornborrow, J. and Coates, J. (eds) (2005). *The sociolinguistics of narrative*. Amsterdam/Philadelphia, PA: J. Benjamins Pub. Co.

Wikan, U. (2000). With life in one's lap: the story of an eye/i (or two). In: Mattingly, C. and Garro, L.C. (eds) *Narrative and the cultural construction of illness and healing*, pp. 212–36. Berkeley, CA: University of California Press.

Woods, A. (2011). The limits of narrative: provocations for the medical humanities. *Medical Humanities*, *37*, 73–8.

Chapter 6

Using focus groups to understand experiences of health and illness

Jenny Kitzinger

Introduction

A focus group is a qualitative method of data collection involving group discussion around a specific experience or issue. When deployed to understand experience of health and illness the group might, for example, focus on participants' experience of a specific illness (e.g. diabetes), caring responsibility (e.g. looking after a brain-injured family member), or procedure (e.g. a particular investigation or operation). Focus groups have been used to study people's experiences of illness, their perceptions of different health behaviours, and to address issues such as how health promotion interventions might work or service delivery be best organized (Frankland and Bloor, 1999; Green and Hart, 1999; Kitzinger, 2005).

The rationale behind talking to research participants in groups rather than a one-to-one interview is that interaction within the group can help to generate a different type of participation. Some people might be more willing to contribute to the research in a group setting and, even more importantly, the group context may generate a different type of conversation than a one-to-one session with a researcher. A defining feature of focus group research is that interaction between participants helps to involve participants and generate ideas as members of the group talk to, question, and react to one another. The key issue in focus group research is to treat such interaction as an integral part of the data (Kitzinger, 1994, p. 103).

Focus groups can be a powerful stand-alone method, or can be used to complement other approaches. For example, combining focus groups with ethnographic work or interviews may access different aspects of people's experience, or even encourage different participants to become involved in the research (Baker and Hinton, 1999) and a focus groups can be used before, or after, a survey to test out a questionnaire design, help explore the meaning of survey results, or to design a more sensitive study in a difficult and emotive area of research (Kitzinger, 1994; Tomlinson et al., 2006).

Designing and conducting a focus group study

Research questions suitable for focus group study

Focus group research is particularly appropriate when the interviewer wishes to encourage participants to explore issues of importance to them, in their own vocabulary, generating their own questions, and pursuing their own priorities—particularly reflecting on some experience they have in common. When group dynamics work well, participants act as co-researchers, taking the research in new and perhaps unexpected directions.

There is no topic that is, by definition, inappropriate for focus group work. Even very 'private' issues can be successfully discussed. The method has been used to explore experiences of death (Kendall et al., 2007), end-of-life decision-making (Tomlinson et al., 2006), and sex (Frith, 2000). Indeed, group work can actively facilitate the discussion of such topics because co-participants can provide mutual support in expressing feelings that might be considered 'deviant'. Participants may report that hearing others talk about their experiences made them less distressed by some of their own reactions or helped them to articulate feelings they had not expressed before. Group work may also make participants feel less isolated. For example, a focus group study with families of severely brain-injured relatives found that people were enthusiastic about meeting each other and participants asked for follow-on discussions to be organized so the conversations could continue. One partici- pant commented later:

> the original focus group—that's been really useful to me, because the sense I had was that I was unusual in asking for things or saying things [...] [and] it knocks you out to be isolated as unusual, [...] it's also like the system locks you in to—'you're the family over there, you're in a family over there, you're another family over there' [...] there's been no suggestion that actually there's value in families [...] having conversations with each other. (Family member of a woman in a vegetative state in conversation with author.)

The focus group is often seen as a relatively empowering data collection tech- nique and is popular in 'action' or feminist research, although this empower- ing or 'participatory' nature cannot be taken for granted (Baker and Hinton, 1999; Wilkinson, 1999). It is critical to be sensitive to the fact that power dynamics can play out within groups and that self-disclosure can pose risks to participants. Rather than pre-judging what is appropriate to explore in group work, attention to the group dynamics and self-censorship within sessions can be an crucial part of the research analysis and strategies can be adopted to mitigate the problem too (see 'Silences and policing in groups' section).

Selecting participants

The focus group will usually bring together people with some type of shared experience, in a non-hierarchical relationship. A size of between four and eight allows for rich discussion. The group members may already know each other, or be strangers—there are pros and cons to either composition. You should also consider the ethical and pragmatic questions regarding whether you want to bring together people at the same 'stage' of experience or not (e.g. early after a cancer diagnosis versus five years postoperative). Even when you have strict recruitment criteria you may find that someone ends up in the group who does not 'qualify'. For example, when I was running focus groups in a hospital unit for the elderly my focus was on *long*-term residents. However, a short-term stay resident participated in one discussion. This proved invaluable—the resident who was soon due to return home prompted far more critical discussion in this group than in those composed entirely of longer-term residents who adopted a more resigned and institutionalized attitude. Many years later, doing research on what relatives wanted from long-care provision for their family members a similar 'mistake' occurred. The sample was supposed to exclude anyone whose relative was only in for respite care—but the inclusion of one such participant by accident proved useful—as he highlighted his needs to learn caring skills from the professionals (e.g. by being involved in physiotherapy sessions) and the different needs of this client group.

Whatever your sampling criteria, it is necessary to be aware how this will limit access to diverse perspectives and who you are *excluding* because of the method of data collection adopted. For example, in a study of people with neurological injuries and diseases simply relying on focus groups would have excluded the perspective of people with certain types of physical impairment—a one-to-one interview was essential to include the voice of a resident on a ventilator who needed frequent rests and interventions such as suctioning during the course of the interview (see Latchem and Kitzinger, 2012). See also Chapters 5 and 13.

Recruitment and location

Recruitment follows usual protocol of providing relevant information to potential participants but has some additional challenges because of the nature of the method. The fact that the focus group usually involves travel to a common venue means that researchers need to provide good directions, offer to reimburse travel expenses, and should over-recruit as some people may not turn up on the day. It often helps attendance if the research session is held at a time and place familiar to participants. Like any good host the facilitator should try to ensure people feel comfortable and welcome. Think carefully about venue (e.g. access, noise levels, privacy, and the different expectations established depending on whether the group meets in a community centre, school, university, hospital, or home).

The facilitator

It is useful to reflect on the persona of the facilitator. In the study of residents in neuro-specialist care settings we made choices to decide which data collection sessions would be conducted by clinical members of the team and which by the outside researcher (who was also a relative of a resident). Each decision took into account the need for the skills of the facilitator/interviewer (e.g. their skill and experience in being able to understand what someone was saying if they had severe speech impediments), the prior relationship involved (e.g. avoiding clinicians collecting data from their own clients), and the way they might be seen by research participants. In this project, the outside researcher also had her own experience of having a loved one with severe brain damage and this was noted as positive by participants (see Latchem and Kitzinger, 2012). One participant in this research project, for example, commented that it felt better to discuss the issue 'with someone who is in the same boat unlike some social worker who has no concept of what life is like at all'. This echoes some of the advantages of using peer researchers in inclusive research (see Chapter 13).

Facilitating discussion

The focus group should not be simply a 'group interview' where people take turn to answer the same question—but a more fluid discussion in which participants are encouraged to talk to one another. The researcher does, however, act as group facilitator or 'host': taking responsibility for arranging the group, offering up initial questions, and supporting the flow of the discussion. The discussion often follows a 'V' funnel-shape—the facilitator initiating discussion via very open questions, and only narrowing to specific prompts later in the session if necessary. For example, examining people's experience of living in long-term care might start with general questions about what is important to *them* and let the discussion flow from that, rather than asking residents to talk about criteria pre-defined by the researcher or the care providers as likely to be important.

Because the facilitator is outnumbered, s/he may sometimes feel s/he has 'lost control' of the topic focus—this can be a challenge, but is not always a bad thing. For example, in a focus groups about care home provision for brain-injured relatives it may be difficult to keep family members focused on care home provision—instead they may first wish to talk at length about the trauma of the original accident and encounters with intensive care, struggles with bureaucracy, and their fears about future funding. This is all integral to these families' experiences and helps to shape their engagement with care home provision and should not be ignored simply because they do not fit with the researchers' (or research funders') predefined focus for the research (Latchem and Kitzinger, 2012).

Prompts and participatory exercises

Object, images, or *texts* are sometimes used in focus groups to help trigger and focus discussion—when researching people's health experiences these could include an advert (e.g. promoting health behaviours), a newspaper article, some images, or objects associated with the issue under discussion (e.g. a diabetic injection kit or a speculum). In one focus group about breast cancer, for example, a participant spontaneously passed round her breast prosthesis, generating fascinating data (see Wilkinson, 1999). Group exercises can also be an innovative way of engaging participants—these might involve story-telling (e.g. adapting the techniques discussed in Chapter 7), producing their own campaign materials (e.g. to challenge stigma), or even something as simple as inviting participants to draw a picture to represent some aspect of their experience. At the end of the focus groups discussing residential care, participants were asked to draw pictures representing 'good' and 'bad' care. These sometimes highlighted issues that had not been mentioned in the verbal discussion. One mother, for example, drew a picture of 'bad care' which showed a figure with a stethoscope giving her daughter drugs without any discussion with the family. The depiction of her daughter (a tiny stick figure in a wheel chair) makes her look very small and vulnerable; her parents are isolated figures to one side of the page. This mother's drawing of 'good care', by contrast, placed her daughter in the centre of the picture, within the symbol of a heart, surrounded by a team of people (with nothing to signal hierarchy or differentiation). As this woman explained, really 'good care' meant her daughter being surrounded by love and good communication, and was only possible if family members were acknowledged as a key part of the care team. (see www.cardiff.ac.uk/jomec/resources/Long_Term_Care.pdf<http://www.cardiff.ac.uk/jomec/resources/Long_Term_Care.pdf>, page 67) This prompted a new topic of discussion that had not previously been part of the focus group—the way in which family members could be excluded from input into medical decision-making on behalf of their loved ones—even if they may have been the key decision-maker for years while a young person was growing up, or had known them before their accident, and thus knew a great deal about the person's medical condition and reactions (e.g. allergies) or about their prior expressed views (e.g. whether or not they would want efforts to resuscitate them in the event on a cardiac arrest).

Silences and policing in groups

Focus group facilitators sometimes find that there can be self-censorship within a group or policing by other group members. This can be seen as a problem or a 'failed' focus group, but it is also possible to analyse silence and silencing itself as a highly significant form of interaction. For example, the sessions I ran with people in long-term hospital residential care for the elderly were designed to explore what they wanted from residential care and what they would like to see improved. For some participants the main research question was itself rather threatening. Participants sometimes commented that there was 'no point' thinking about what they disliked about their current situation. In the course of discussion it was evident that these boundaries were established in reaction to their limited choices and an element of self-censorship was used to manage hope, and therefore disappointment. In addition to this, elderly people in residential care were clearly acutely aware of being a captive population living under highly circumscribed conditions. Some residents even tried to prevent others from criticizing staff (see Kitzinger and Farquhar, 1999). Similar evidence of policing from other group members was evident in a group discussion with young women about infant feeding. This discussion took place within a community where breastfeeding was very unusual—all the young women in the group were formula-feeding their babies, apart from one who was in the late stages of pregnancy and was considering breastfeeding. When this young woman expressed interest in breastfeeding other members of the group underlined their disgust at breastfeeding in public, suggested that her boyfriend was only supportive because he wanted to be able to look at her breasts more often, and disputed her suggestions of health benefits ('If it is going to get asthma it is going to get asthma'). They also mocked this young woman's stance ('She just wants to be different') and made comments such as: 'You end up bottle-feeding anyway'.

Such interactions illustrate how groups may induce conformity to group norms or a shared resistance to outside pressure. Focus groups can illustrate such peer group pressure and may also serve as an arena in which new definitions are formed drawing on common (but not previously shared) experiences and building new frameworks for understanding (Dahlin-Ivanoff and Hultberg, 2006). This was a striking feature in some of the discussions I have conducted addressing sexual harassment and violence—for example, discussion of childhood sexual abuse in the 1980s when such experiences were very hidden and socially unrecognized (for examples of such transformation see Kitzinger and Farquhar, 1999).

A researcher needs to be aware of how participants can censor themselves or each other and can approach this issue in three ways: documenting and analysing such processes; seeking to help a group overcome self-policing; or circumventing this by, for example, offering people the option of writing down any comments or talk to the facilitator one-to-one after the group.

Problem solving in focus groups

Inviting participants to reflect on their shared experience together may lead to participants doing some of the 'work' to interpret shared needs or consider potential improvements in their common situation. For example, research participants may shift from self-blaming explanations ('I'm stupid not to have understood what the doctor was telling me') to the exploration of structural solutions ('If we've *all* felt confused about what we've been told maybe it would help if we could take away a tape-recording of the consultation?'). Even if they do not come up with 'solutions' they may unpack and explore some of the problems. Discussions between young/middle-aged adults with neurological illnesses (such as multiple sclerosis) highlighted the tensions they have to manage in their day-to-day lives in a neurology long-term care centre. Residents reflected on the 'rules' about going out alone and the tension between safety and making their own risk judgements. Lively debate was also triggered when reflecting on how to manage their own well-being while also maintaining a sense of community in a centre which included residents with brain injuries which could make them 'disruptive'. When one resident suggested that it might be best to put all the 'screamers and shouters' in one corridor, because 'When you've got something like MS you need some peace and quiet', another wondered if that would be 'discrimination' and commented: 'I've heard some families say "oh it's not right you, you people being amongst people like that", like "that", as if people with a head injury shouldn't be looked at, as if it's so monstrous to see them, like we should be shielded and protected from looking at that. We shouldn't have to hear people shouting all day but then…' (Latchem and Kitzinger, 2012).

Recording the data

It is ideal to audio record the session because, as should be clear from some of the extracts already quoted, a great deal of data would be lost if the researcher simply relied on taking notes. Some researchers like to video record groups in order to capture non-verbal communication (see also Chapter 4). People often forget the presence of cameras, although they can be inhibiting for some participants, so if systematic analysis of such non-verbal interactions is not essential then it is usually reasonable simply to note any striking non-verbal behaviours at the time. It is also useful to take notes during the session (unless you have a very agile brain and keen memory) as discussion may be so rich you may want an aide-memoire to come back to towards the end of the group. Ideally discussions are fully transcribed—this is a very long process, allow at least four hours to transcribe every hour of discussion. For most projects a simplified transcription is sufficient, but for some projects, such as those adopting 'conversation analysis', specialist skills are needed (systematically recording false starts, length of all pauses, emphasis on different syllables, etc.).

Analysing and presenting findings

The talk in the focus group can be treated in diverse ways. Often researchers simply present a systematic analysis of key themes, alongside ensuring that the diversity of voices is represented. It is also useful to go beyond the surface 'content' of the discussion and researchers should reflect on how people interact and communicate with one another and acknowledge that 'focus groups are social spaces in which participants co-construct the "patient's view" by sharing, contesting and acquiring knowledge' (Lehoux et al., 2006, p. 2091). How far you pursue this as a *focus* of analysis may depend on your theoretical perspective and research objectives but some consideration of such aspects can be useful for any project. For example:

- Attention to when participants support or undermine one another in a focus group study of infant feeding practice highlighted the operation of social pressure within the group sessions (see earlier example).

- Attention to the operation of anecdotes in a study of public understanding of AIDS highlighted how stigma was reinforced through the deployment of urban myths about the 'vengeful AIDS carrier' (Kitzinger, 1994).

- Attention to 'sensitive moments' in the discussion on childhood sexual abuse highlighted the marking of cultural norms and taboos (Kitzinger and Farquhar, 1999).

Other researchers have looked at the deployment of humour within focus groups, or systematically approached the analysis through the lens of conversation analysis or the study of 'talk' (Myers and Macnaghten, 1999; Frith, 2000) (see Chapter 4).

Limitations and final reflections

The focus group will not be the ideal method of data collection for every project. It can be time consuming to set up and difficult to generate lively discussion in some cases, which can be dispiriting. The nature of group discussion also means that you are unlikely to elicit the depth of personal narrative that can be generated in interview (see Chapter 5). It can be difficult to track individual voices and, if people cut across each other, as they will do in any lively discussion, this may leave tantalizing, and frustrating, unfinished sentences hanging in the air. The data can also be cumbersome to present. It can fall between stools by failing to allow the researcher to extract individual 'opinions' or try to tabulate 'attitudes' (in the style of the survey) but also lacking the 'storytelling' appeal of an extract from an interview (e.g. Chapter 7). This does not mean that focus group data are inferior. On the contrary, the fluid nature of group discussion may actually challenge both the apparently 'objective' knowledge obtained from surveys and the illusion of the pure authentic narrative sometimes implied in the presentation of interview material. Focus group data resist the 'context-stripping' of talk, and isolation of individual opinions or stories as if they can be told cut off from relationships with others (Wilkinson, 1999, p. 65). Focus group work lends itself to thinking of talk as a performance and examining how stances are adopted, knowledge mobilized, and ideas negotiated in the group context. It also can reflect the way in which understandings are formed, and decisions made in personal partnerships and within the context of broader communities in a particular time and place. Indeed, the most troublesome aspects of focus groups—the dialogical, context-bound, culturally sensitive, unstable, and collective nature of the discussion—could be the grit that makes the pearl in this methodological oyster. To finish by mixing metaphors, however, let me also promote mixing methods and adopting the approach of 'horses for courses'. All the approaches outlined in this volume have potential for exploring and using different aspects of experience—experimenting with any of these methods to see what it might add to a project, could be an exciting and useful part of developing the research design or contextualizing and reflecting on the findings.

Further reading

Barbour, R. (2008). *Doing focus groups (qualitative research kit)*. London: Sage.

Barbour, R. and Kitzinger, J. (eds) (1999). *Developing focus group research: Politics, theory and practice*. London: Sage.

Bloor, M., *et al.* (2001). *Focus groups in social research*. London: Sage.

Stewart, D., Shamdasani, P., and Rook, D. (2007). *Focus groups: Theory and practice*. London: Sage.

References

Baker, R. and Hinton, R. (1999). Do focus groups facilitate meaningful participation in social research? In: Barbour, R. and Kitzinger, J. (eds) *Developing focus group research: Politics, theory and practice*, pp. 79–98. London: Sage.

Dahlin-Ivanoff, S. and Hultberg, J. (2006). Understanding the multiple realities of everyday life: Basic assumptions in focus-group methodology. *Scandinavian Journal of Occupational Therapy*, 13(2), 125–32.

Frankland, J. and Bloor, M. (1999). Some issues arising in the systematic analysis of focus group materials. In: Barbour, R. and Kitzinger, J. (eds) *Developing focus group research: Politics, theory and practice*, pp. 144–55. London: Sage.

Frith, H. (2000). Focusing on sex: using focus groups in sex research. *Sexualities*, 3, 275–97.

Green, J. and Hart, L. (1999). Combining focus groups and interviews: telling how it is; telling how it feels. In: Barbour, R. and Kitzinger, J. (eds) *Developing focus group research: Politics, theory and practice*, pp. 21–35. London: Sage.

Kendall, M., *et al.* (2007). Key challenges and ways forward in researching the 'good death': qualitative in-depth interview and focus group study. *British Medical Journal*, 334, 521–4.

Kitzinger, J. (1994). The methodology of focus groups: the importance of interactions between research participants. *Sociology of Health and Illness*, 16, 103–21.

Kitzinger, J. (2005). Focus group research: using group dynamics to explore perceptions, experiences and understandings. In: Holloway, I. (ed.) *Qualitative research in health care*. pp. 56–69. Maidenhead: Open University Press.

Kitzinger, J. and Farquhar, C. (1999). The analytical potential of 'sensitive moments' in focus group discussions. In: Barbour, R. and Kitzinger, J. (eds) *Developing focus group research: Politics, theory and practice*, pp. 156–72. London: Sage.

Latchem, J. and Kitzinger, J. (2012). *What is important to residents with neurological conditions and their relatives in rehabilitation and long-term care centres?* Research Report, Cardiff University. Available at: <http://www.cardiff.ac.uk/jomec/resources/Long_Term_Care.pdf>.

Lehoux, P., Poland, B., and Daudelin, G. (2006). Focus group research and 'the patient's view' *Social Science & Medicine*, 63(8), 2091–104.

Myers, G. and Macnaghten, P. (1999). Can focus groups be analyzed as talk? In: Barbour R. and Kitzinger, J. (eds) *Developing focus group research: Politics, theory and practice*, pp. 173–85. London: Sage.

Tomlinson, D., *et al.* (2006). Parental decision making in pediatric cancer end-of-life care: using focus group methodology as a pre-phase to seek participant design input. *European Journal of Oncology Nursing, 10,* 198–206.

Wilkinson, S. (1999). How useful are focus groups in feminist research? In: Barbour, R. and Kitzinger, J. (eds) *Developing focus group research: Politics, theory and practice.* pp. 64–78. London: Sage.

Chapter 7

Story gathering: collecting and analysing spontaneously-shared stories as research data

Trisha Greenhalgh

Background

Stories are rich research data, but the stories people tell in formal research interviews differ from those told spontaneously in real life. Collecting stories in 'naturalistic' settings has both strengths and limitations (see 'Discussion'). In this chapter, we describe a new approach to naturalistic story gathering using diabetes self-management as a worked example.

We make sense of our lives by retrospectively and prospectively 'storying' our experiences (Bruner, 1990). Stories are defined by chronology (unfolding over time), characters, setting, trouble, and plot (Aristotle, 1996). In illness narratives, 'trouble' comprises pain, disability, disfigurement, loss of independence, and so on (Frank, 1995). Coping with chronic illness and minimizing its impact requires sense-making and biographical work (Strauss, 1975). In cross-cultural illness narratives, personal experience is nested within a wider narrative of personal, family, and community—which for the immigrant patient may include displacement, loss of social status, economic hardship, and perhaps discrimination following immigration.

A 'textbook' narrative is structurally coherent with a beginning, middle, and ending, but real-world narratives may emerge as a bricolage of incomplete, inconsistent story fragments (Riessman, 2008). Stories are image rich, action-packed, and laden with emotions—hence are potentially powerful vehicles for educational messages (McDrury and Alterio, 2002).

Whilst narratives have often been used to explore illness from the patient's perspective, there are far fewer examples of such narratives being used to inform a grounded and nuanced approach to patient education. The question arises: how can we provide education that is useful and meaningful to people with a condition unless we know how that condition affects both their identity and the practicalities of daily life for them? Yet as policy in chronic disease management shifts from a focus on episodic, clinician-led care to one that emphasizes self-management, the importance of understanding the patient narrative increases.

'Self-management' is a contested term—referring (in different literatures) to particular behaviours and lifestyles; coping emotionally and practically with illness; participating in illness-related networks and social movements; and challenging inadequate provision of services (Hinder and Greenhalgh, 2012). In the study which forms the basis of the example in this chapter, we sought to explore the stories told (and enacted) by people with diabetes and use these stories to design self-management education and support.

Our research questions included: (1) what stories do people from minority ethnic groups in socio-economically deprived areas tell about their diabetes and efforts to live with it? and (2) how can these stories inform the design of culturally congruent self-management programmes?

The 'naturalistic story-gathering' approach

Building on earlier work to develop and validate a group-based story-sharing intervention (Greenhalgh et al., 2005), and as part of a randomized controlled trial to test that intervention (Greenhalgh et al., 2011a, 2011b), we collected stories shared in peer support groups held in six different ethnic languages. The study was based in a deprived and ethnically diverse part of London with high diabetes prevalence. Eighty-two people had been referred for diabetes education and randomized to story-sharing groups. They ranged in age from 25 to 82 years; 20 were on insulin and 22 were male. All were first- or second-generation immigrants from African Caribbean (seven participants), Bangladeshi (23), Tamil (11), Punjabi/Urdu (34), and Somali (seven) communities. Each group was homogeneous for language and ethnicity (with some overlap of Pubjabi and Urdu), but mixed gender (though groups sometimes spontaneously split into men and women for discussions of gender-sensitive topics).

Because our early research had identified informal stories (such as gossip or hearsay) told by an equal-status peer (as opposed to 'standardized' or 'expert' accounts) as the trigger for behaviour change (Greenhalgh et al., 1998), the intervention was intentionally unstructured and informal, and didactic teaching by staff was strongly discouraged. Following Hawe et al. (2004), we recognized that complex interventions may include flexibility in application in different settings yet must have well-defined core components. These were:

◆ Sessions must involve spontaneous, informal, and unstructured story sharing (participants should be encouraged to tell whatever stories they want about their condition, in whatever order, with no stipulation of what is 'important' or 'legitimate').

- Sessions must be facilitated non-directively by a non-clinical professional or volunteer trained in the sharing stories model.
- Input of clinical professionals (doctors, nurses, dieticians, etc.) must be in the form of a response to the stories shared by group participants.

In practice, the groups were run as follows. Each group had ten to 12 participants; sessions lasted around two hours (the venue was booked for three hours to allow for a 'social time' and to accommodate late arrivals); they were held two-weekly for six months.

Participants were encouraged to identify a theme for a forthcoming session, which was typically a topic that had emerged in discussion the previous session (e.g. 'feeding the family', 'medication', 'dealing with doctors'). They were asked to bring personal stories on the agreed topic next time, and the principle of participant-led, story-based topic discussions was followed as far as possible.

On arrival, participants had ten to 15 minutes (sometimes more) 'social time' before being asked to get into 'buzz groups' of two to three and share their stories. After about 20 minutes, the facilitator invited them to regroup in a plenary format and asked 'Does any group have a good story to share?'. This often allowed a story with important learning points to emerge, after being 'tried out' in the safety of the buzz group. Informal discussion on this story was encouraged, with a focus on the practicalities and moral challenges that the story raised. Whilst the generic design for the group session was around the 'told story', in practice many stories were enacted with visual 'props'—for example, pills are often passed round when discussing medication; or samples of rice when discussing glycaemic index. If stories prompted action (e.g. stories about exercise prompted the group to try out chair-based or stretching exercises), this was encouraged.

Thus, each story-sharing group was led by a bilingual health advocate (BHA) with some input from a clinician—most usually a diabetes specialist nurse but depending on the chosen session topic, a chiropodist, dietician, general practitioner (GP), pharmacist, or physical trainer was invited to attend either as well as, or instead of, the nurse. The BHA facilitated the group in a non-directive manner, encouraging the sharing of personal stories about diabetes and its impact, which s/he interpreted and invited the health professional to comment on. The BHA sought to work actively with the health professional to ensure that the focus of discussion was on 'explaining why X happened in the story' rather than 'giving a talk on X'.

To capture the stories, we used quasi-naturalistic story gathering (collecting naturally-occurring talk during real social interaction), though groups were not strictly naturalistic since they were set up as part of a trial.

Members of the research team attended a total of 65 group sessions. We sat in the group circle and made field notes on group dynamics, issues discussed, emotions displayed and actions observed, which we typed up immediately afterwards. To be captured, stories had to be translated by the facilitator without interrupting the group discussion or spontaneously retold in English by a group member. This required the researcher to exercise flexibility and judgement, not least because—as in any multilingual group where informal stories are being shared—the narratives overlapped; different fragments of the narrative were sometimes told in different languages; and each narrative attracted a response and/or a counter-narrative (that is, a story which illustrated the opposite point to the one being made in a previous story). There was no self-evident or technical way for the researcher to decide which stories to record in a notebook or which to ask the BHA or another group member to translate in real time. Rather, we used the narrative 'tool' of simple curiosity, selecting those stories that surprised, intrigued, delighted, or shocked us.

Analysing naturalistic narratives

Stories can be analysed as pieces of text (for example, the researcher could go through a printed story with a highlighter pen and mark up particular words or phrases, but take no account of the narrative features such as whether the story is a 'comedy' or a 'tragedy', who the 'heroes' and 'villains', are and what constitutes the 'plot'), and/or they can be analysed *as literature* with attention to all these features and more. In particular, a narrative analysis goes beyond the text itself and asks questions about the narrator and the act of narrating.

In our example, we undertook a preliminary thematic analysis mainly to gain familiarity with the data. For this, we used Ritchie and Spencer's framework method to chart data on a spreadsheet and iteratively refine a taxonomy of issues raised (Ritchie and Lewis, 2003). In a subsequent, more detailed, narrative analysis, we identified stories or story fragments and for each one identified, we considered literary features such temporality, characterization, contextualization, and emplotment (e.g. how events and actions were juxtaposed in a particular way to imply motive or causality). We also considered the context in which a particular story was told, the narrator's (sometimes urgent) desire to tell this story to the group, and the reciprocal desire of the audience to hear it, participate in its interpretation, and contribute to its resolution. To achieve this, we drew on Bakhtin's dialogical approach and Riessman's notion of storytelling as performance (Bakhtin, 1981; Riessman, 2008).

Thus, our interpretive analysis took account of both the product of storytelling (narrative as noun) and its process (narrative as verb).

The messy and heterogeneous nature of narrative data

The researcher who seeks to collect a tidy set of 'textbook' stories from naturalistic story gathering, each with a clear beginning, middle, and end, will be disappointed. As suggested earlier, narratives shared in groups come in many different shapes and sizes, and are not infrequently incomplete. The messy nature of the data may be further compounded by the lack of verbatim recordings (for example, if many stories are told in quick succession the researcher may capture only parts of some of them).

Many 'stories' captured in our handwritten field notes of the group sessions were thus short and fragmentary, and some were offered in response to another fragment on the same topic told by another participant (hence could only meaningfully be analysed in conjunction with those fragments). Other stories were longer and had a more definitive narrative structure; these sometimes became the focus of the day's meeting with the facilitator and other participants asking further questions, which shaped the unfolding narrative. Some longer narratives (e.g. a person's efforts to get a referral from a reluctant GP) became recurring topics in successive meetings, with the narrator offering (or being asked for) an update by the group. Some topics (e.g. efforts to lose weight) began as one person's story but became collectivized as other group members offered similar or contrasting ones.

Occasionally, a narrator would claim the floor by standing up or presenting an artefact (e.g. a hospital letter or packet of tablets) and offering a story about this. Many stories were presented emotionally—with laughter, tears, or apparent anger. These contrast markedly with the fictional vignettes or images typically given in educational materials, in which self-managing patients are depicted somewhat blandly as doing context-independent tasks such as 'eating healthily' or 'exercising'. In contrast, real-life accounts depict the work of self-management as having *social meaning* and *moral worth*. Indeed, this was why they came across as stories, however fragmentary, and why group members chose to afford significance to them.

Finding 'storylines' in narrative data

Every story is unique, but at a higher level of abstraction several stories may share a common thread or 'storyline'. A challenge in analysing a large dataset

of naturalistic stories is to identify these storylines and reflect on their implications (see Chapter 5).

Our preliminary 'framework' analysis revealed seven self-management
challenges facing the person with diabetes: knowledge, diet, exercise,
medication, foot care, self-monitoring, and attending check-ups. These map
closely to the domains covered by previous studies of diabetes knowledge,
and to self-management education guidelines (Funnell et al., 2009). But an
important finding of the study was that these challenges were never presented
purely as 'tasks' but were framed within particular storylines, which were
common to all cultural groups studied. Next, we describe two of these
storylines in detail to illustrate the point that storylines add much to the
research findings *over and above* the specific topics talked about. The other
six storylines are illustrated briefly in Table 7.1 and presented in more detail
elsewhere (Greenhalgh et al., 2011b).

Storyline 1: becoming sick

> (I was) panicky, fear gripped me...I didn't think I would die but I was very
> frightened—I had heard about diabetes in the family. I cried for 3 days because I was
> frightened and everyone said to me awful things would happen to me, strokes and
> I don't know what...I am still frightened. (Participant in Tamil group, T1.)

In all of the groups, the first session was spontaneously spent with each participant in turn describing the experience of diagnosis. Most had felt shock,
feelings of hopelessness, loss, and isolation—reactions which link to Frank's
notion of 'deep illness', affecting all life choices and decisions (Frank, 1995).
Many told stories of others who had developed terrible complications (e.g.
amputation) and anticipated that they would too. Some people revealed fear
of stigma, ill-defined fears, and/or specific knowledge gaps. One of the com-
monest questions was whether to conceal or share the news of the diagnosis,
and with whom.

Storyline 2: becoming a practitioner of self-management

> They [various tablets for diabetes] are like a herd of cattle for me and I remember
> each one like a different cow. (Participant recently immigrated from Somalia where
> she had lived a nomadic life herding cattle, group S4.)

Around half of all the stories exchanged in the groups involved either seeking
or providing tacit knowledge relating to diet, physical activity, self-monitoring,
and managing medication, thereby operationalizing self-management within
the social and practical constraints of their daily lives. Strategies employed
were often grounded in particular cultural symbols or gender roles, but the

Table 7.1 How the findings from a diabetes story-gathering study informed diabetes self-management education

Storyline	Implication for education
1. Becoming sick Participants who have not come to terms with the diagnosis may not engage with self-management	People should have an opportunity to tell 'the story of my illness'
2. Rebuilding spoiled identity Moving on from the diagnosis involves biographical work linked to practical actions	Educators should understand how physical and practical measures can help identity-rebuilding
3. Becoming a practitioner of self-management Self-management is learnt partly through watching, listening, and building social networks	Educators should promote tacit knowledge exchange through stories
4. Living a disciplined and balanced life Many great religions uphold the principles of diabetes self-management: looking after the body, resisting excess and indolence, and observing rituals	Programmes should reflect the fact that some people make sense of their lives through religion
5. Mobilizing a care network The 'self-managing' patient is usually sited in a care network comprising family, community, and health professionals	Input from family and peers should be supported flexibly
6. Navigating and negotiating in the healthcare system Access barriers and power differentials can hamper diabetes management	Programmes should address accessing healthcare and communicating with staff
7. Managing the micro-morality of lifestyle choices Self-management often poses small-scale moral choices, especially how to spend limited family income	Educators should draw on stories to explore moral dilemmas
8. Taking collective action Stories may be enacted by the group as well as told orally. Enacted stories have great potential to energize and motivate.	Educators should recognize and support the 'social drama' aspects of group work

Reproduced with permission from Greenhalgh, T. et al. New models of self-management education for minority ethnic groups: pilot randomized trial of a story-sharing intervention. *Journal of Health Services Research and Policy*, Volume 16, Number 1, pp. 28–36, January 2012, Copyright © The Royal Society of Medicine Press Ltd, UK, DOI: 10.1258/jhsrp.2010.009159.

task of 'becoming a practitioner' was a common challenge for all. Talk about the practicalities of self-management was led by a few experienced members in each group, but others joined in with time. For example, a man who had recently been widowed kept quiet for several sessions whenever the subject of shopping or cooking came up, but eventually he began to tell stories about trying out recipes learnt from the women in the group.

The exchange of tacit knowledge through stories resonated with Lave and Wenger's notion of community of practice—an informal group in which learning is not about amassing socially disembodied facts but about 'legitimate peripheral participation' (watching, listening, developing an identity through practice, and building the social networks that form the scaffolding for tacit knowledge acquisition) (Lave and Wenger, 1991).

Application of naturalistic story gathering

It is worth reflecting on what this novel approach (which produced a messy and difficult-to-analyse dataset) achieved over and above what might have been achieved through more conventional qualitative research (such as one-to-one semi-structured interviews or focus groups). By collecting and analysing narratives from people with diabetes from minority ethnic groups in a deprived part of London, we confirmed previous biomedical research on knowledge and skills needed for self-management (Funnell et al., 2009) and the sociological notion of illness narrative as biographical work (Strauss, 1975; Bury, 1985). We also made a number of original contributions both to the clinical literature on diabetes and to the methodology of narrative research.

Cross-cultural research traditionally seeks to identify and explain differences between ethnic or social groups. One of the most striking findings in this study was the common storylines occurring in all the groups despite a wide range of different cultural backgrounds, religions, and the inclusion of both first- and second-generation immigrants. We found that commonalities across groups, especially the triple jeopardy of immigrant status, material poverty, and low functional health literacy, were more striking than the differences between them.

By synthesizing these overarching storylines into a more-or-less holistic picture of what it is to live with diabetes, we were able to draw a closer link between biomedical and sociological research on self-management of chronic illness. Previous literature on this topic had been somewhat polarized, considering *either* the biomedical skill set (can the patient demonstrate diabetes knowledge and perform particular self-management tasks?) *or* the illness narrative (can the person make sense of their illness, restore coherence and balance in their life and address moral questions?) (Greenhalgh, 2009). Through naturalistic story gathering followed by an explicitly *narrative* analysis of the dataset, we concluded that these two perspectives are not incommensurable but two sides of the same coin: behaviours expected of the self-managing patient come to be applied in practice by being included within particular illness storylines which give them meaning and purpose.

The study allowed us to refine a complex intervention for education and peer support in minority ethnic groups with diabetes (Table 7.1).

An individual's ability to manage their diabetes is largely unrelated to their level of factual knowledge, a finding that confirms other work in low-literacy minority ethnic groups (von Goeler et al., 2003; Carbone et al., 2007; Tang et al., 2008). Participants appeared to recognize the distinction between abstract knowledge ('knowing-that'), which they said they gained from health professionals, and tacit or practical understanding ('knowing-how'), which they felt they gained from sharing stories. One participant put it like this: 'We learn the facts from you [health professionals] but we learn the meaning and how to do things from one another'.

Naturalistic story gathering has potential to inform a radical new curriculum for patient education and support. The approach may be particularly pertinent when the patient's 'real life' includes hardship, material constraints, and barriers of language and literacy.

Our findings suggested the need for two radical developments in the design and delivery of self-management education for people with chronic illness. First, programmes should be oriented more explicitly towards capturing and bearing witness to the overarching storylines through which the experience of chronic illness, and the work of self-management, is patterned. Importantly, these storylines are discernible when stories are told informally and spontaneously. Second, diabetes education should be more firmly grounded in the pedagogical distinction between know-that knowledge (easy to codify and standardize) and know-how knowledge (tacit, applied, and context-specific, hence impossible to codify or standardize). 'Structured' self-management education will cover only the former (Funnell et al., 2009); sharing stories informally is one way of covering the latter.

Strengths and limitations

Naturalistic story gathering has methodological strengths and limitations. Creating an environment in which people feel free to share stories presents challenges to the researcher who wishes both to preserve the naturalism, and record the content of, the encounter. Of course, the very presence of a researcher or health professional (especially perhaps if not from the same ethnic group as the participants) may also influence the nature or format of the stories told.

Our own decision not to record the group sessions was made because, in early pilot work (in which we held 'drop-in' groups for people with diabetes), group members were emphatically opposed to tape recording of the sessions. This may have been because some attenders were illegal immigrants or had other reason to distrust the use of recording equipment. Other researchers may decide to audio or video recording a storytelling group if they feel that they need to transcribe detailed verbatim accounts for data analysis (and translation).

Whatever the chosen approach to capturing stories as research data, there is a trade-off between the authenticity of the story (for example, its informality, spontaneity, and original language) and the accuracy with which it can be recorded—the control exercised by the research participants and the extent to which health researchers are visible in the process. In a multilingual storytelling group the researcher may have to rely on translations (and, sometimes, a re-telling).

However, selective translation (and the fact that the researchers in our study were monolingual) could be seen a positive feature, since it allowed the group to control and even negotiate what was to be shared as 'data'. Our data suggest that people talked very freely when they were assured that the researcher would only hear the stories if they or the BHA chose to translate them.

Conclusion

While this conclusion needs to be confirmed in other studies, we tentatively conclude that naturalistic story gathering may be especially suited to capturing the process by which tacit knowledge is exchanged among peers. Furthermore, the approach led us to a new hypothesis: that 'non-compliance' with self-management tasks is more often linked to a lack of 'know-how' knowledge (a problem for which the exchange of tacit knowledge through stories may offer a solution) or to the ambiguous social meaning and moral worth which particular tasks may hold (a problem for which group negotiation of meaning and morality may offer a solution) than to lack of factual, know-what knowledge.

The empirical study that forms the basis of this chapter illustrates some but almost certainly not all the potential advantages and disadvantages of naturalistic story gathering in clinical research. Many methodological questions (such as the trade-off between recording and not recording stories verbatim, and the use or not of bilingual researchers) remain unanswered. Indeed, it could be argued that these questions are unanswerable in the abstract, since the 'right' method can only be decided in relation to a particular research question, context, sample, and budget. We would be most interested to hear from other health researchers who have used the naturalistic approach in narrative research.

Acknowledgements

We thank group participants for their stories and permission to share and learn from them; clinicians, managers, advocates, and volunteers who participated directly in the study; external advisors who served on our steering group; and the NHSSDO Programme who funded the study.

References

Aristotle (1996). *Poetics*, trans. M. Heath. London, Penguin.

Bakhtin, M. (1981). Discourse in the novel. In: Holquist, M (ed.) *The dialogic imagination. Four essays by M.M. Bakhtin*. Austin, TX: University of Texas Press.

Bruner, J. (1990). *Acts of meaning*. Cambridge, MA: Harvard University Press.

Bury, M. (1985). Chronic illness as biographical disruption. *Sociology of Health and Illness*, 4, 167–82.

Carbone, E.T., *et al.* (2007). Diabetes self-management: perspectives of Latino patients and their health care providers. *Patient Education and Counseling*, 66, 202–10.

Frank, A. (1995). *The wounded storyteller: Body, illness, and ethics*. Chicago, IL: University of Chicago Press.

Funnell, M.M., *et al.* (2009). National standards for diabetes self-management education. *Diabetes Care*, 32(1), 87–94.

Greenhalgh, T. (2009). Patient and public involvement in chronic illness: beyond the expert patient. *British Medical Journal*, 338, 49.

Greenhalgh, T., Helman, C., and Chowdhury, A.M. (1998). Health beliefs and folk models of diabetes in British Bangladeshis: a qualitative study. *British Medical Journal*, 316, 978–83.

Greenhalgh, T., Collard, A., and Begum, N. (2005). Sharing stories: complex intervention for diabetes education in minority ethnic groups who do not speak English. *British Medical Journal*, 330, 628–33.

Greenhalgh, T., *et al.* (2011a). New models of self-management education for minority ethnic groups: pilot randomized trial of a story-sharing intervention. *Journal of Health Services Research and Policy*, 16, 28–36.

Greenhalgh, T., *et al.* (2011b). Storylines of self-management: narratives of people with diabetes from a multiethnic inner city population. *Journal of Health Services Research & Policy*, 16, 37–43.

Hawe, P., Sheill, A., and Riley, B. (2004). Complex interventions: how 'out of control' can a randomised controlled trial be? *British Medical Journal*, 328, 1561–3.

Hinder, S. and Greenhalgh, T. (2012). 'This does my head in'. Ethnographic study of self-management by people with diabetes. *BMC Health Services Research*, 12, 83.

Lave, J. and Wenger, E. (1991). *Situated learning: Legitimate peripheral participation.* Cambridge: Cambridge University Press.

McDrury, J. and Alterio, M. (2002). *Learning through storytelling in higher education: Using reflection and experience to improve learning.* Auckland: Routledge Falmer.

Riessman, C.K. (2008). *Narrative methods for the human sciences.* Thousand Oaks, CA: Sage.

Ritchie, J. and Lewis, J. (2003). *Qualitative research practice.* London: Sage.

Strauss, A.L. (1975). *Chronic illness and the quality of life.* St. Louis, MO: Mosby.

Tang, Y.H., *et al.* (2008). Health literacy, complication awareness, and diabetic control in patients with type 2 diabetes mellitus. *Journal of Advanced Nursing, 62,* 74–83.

Von Goeler, D.S., *et al.* (2003). Self-management of type 2 diabetes: a survey of low-income urban Puerto Ricans. *The Diabetes Educator, 29,* 663–72.

Chapter 8

Patient reported outcomes

Crispin Jenkinson and Ray Fitzpatrick

Introduction

Patient self-reports of their health status and quality of life are increasingly central to the evaluation of healthcare interventions and provision. Patient reported outcome measures (PROMs) are now regularly used to systematically gain meaningful subjective accounts from those receiving care. This is in stark contrast to the prevailing approach adopted to outcomes measurement throughout most of the 20th century and before: namely, that outcomes should be assessed by professionals, such as clinicians and researchers. Reports from patients were, traditionally, viewed as subjective, and consequently unreliable. However, evidence has accumulated that patient reports are not only a reliable source of information, but also one of the most important. This chapter outlines the principles of measurement adopted in this field of research, and the uses to which such information is put in contemporary healthcare.

Measuring patient reported outcomes

Traditionally, evaluation of medical treatment has relied upon measures of morbidity and mortality, whilst medical practitioners have based judgements for intervention on clinical, radiological, and laboratory measures. However, clinically assessed outcomes of treatment do not always reflect those of patients. Over the past few decades the importance of patient-based reports has been recognized (Dawson et al., 2010). The purpose of such evaluation is to provide more meaningful assessments of patient health and the benefits and harms that may result from healthcare (Fitzpatrick et al., 1992). PROMs are questionnaires designed to gain data on aspects of self-reported health, and typically cover topics such as emotional health and functional status. Crucially, they are normally used before and after an intervention and the change between scores is the outcome potentially related to the intervention.

There are a wide variety of applications of health status measures, and the requirements of measures differ across these applications. Some instruments are generic in nature (such as the widely used 36-item Short Form (SF-36) Health Survey, version 2 (Ware, 2007)) and permit comparison with normative values gained from the general population, whilst others are specific to a particular condition or procedure (such as the 39-item Parkinson's Disease Questionnaire (Jenkinson et al., 2012)). Instruments can vary in their scoring, with some providing a profile of scores across a range of areas (e.g. emotional health, social functioning, mobility, etc.) and others a single overall score, whilst some provide both profile and index scores. Some measures can be used in health economic analyses. Before considering the nature of subjective health measures it is worth considering the variety of applications in which data gained directly and systematically from the patient's perspective could be of value.

Applications of health status measures

A number of potential uses have been suggested for PROMs. We will confine ourselves here to the most commonly cited applications, namely as outcomes in randomized controlled trials, routine evaluation and monitoring of healthcare, clinical decision-making, and cost–utility studies.

It is generally agreed that PROMs can play an important role in the evaluation of treatments in randomized controlled trials (Osaba, 2005). PROMs may be measured as either a primary or secondary outcome. For example, in a trial looking at outcomes of treatment for Parkinson's disease the primary outcome was self-reported health status, as measured by the 39-item Parkinson's Disease Questionnaire (Williams et al., 2010). Even when not used as a primary outcome, PRO data can still be influential as secondary outcomes. For example, a trial evaluating a new therapy for recurrent malignant gliomas of the brain compared with an existing treatment found no difference in the primary outcome of survival rates. However, the new treatment was found to perform better in a number of aspects of self-reported health status (Osaba et al., 2000).

Reports on clinical trials incorporating PROMs as primary or secondary end points should, of course, conform to guidelines for reporting any randomized trial, but the rationale for the selection of a particular PROM must be made explicit (Fitzpatrick et al., 1998). The US Food and Drug Administration (FDA) has produced recommendations on the selection and application of PROMs in clinical trials (Food and Drug Administration, 2009). The FDA guidelines state that PROMs selected for inclusion in a trial should have a well-documented developmental history, accessible via peer reviewed publications, and the content of the measure should be based on a clearly documented process of patient interviews with input from experts in the field. There should be evidence of reliability, validity, and, importantly, sensitivity to change of the PRO in the patient group under scrutiny, and differences between groups must be meaningful: statistically significant differences alone may be related to differences so small as to be both subjectively and clinically meaningless.

The idea that PROMs might be used to routinely monitor outcomes was first mooted in the early 1990s (Lansky et al., 1992), but widespread use of routine PROM data collection has been slow to develop. The National Health Service (NHS) in England has recently launched a programme to obtain PROM data from patients undergoing certain elective procedures (Valderas et al., 2012). PROM data has been collected using both condition-specific instruments (such as the Oxford Hip Score for hip replacement (Dawson et al., 1996)) and generic measures (the EuroQol EQ-5D (EuroQol Group, 1990)). More widespread use of PROMs is currently being explored. Some have argued that this type of measurement is essential for future evaluation of healthcare services provided by the NHS (Darzi, 2008). The challenge here is to make the information gained from such surveys meaningful to clinicians and health service managers. Sample sizes must be sufficiently large to permit meaningful comparisons, and adjustments are likely to be necessary to account for potentially confounding characteristics of the patient groups.

PROMs have been suggested as potentially valuable in the clinical interview. Use of PROMs can improve patient–clinician communication, which in turn may contribute to improved outcomes (Valderas et al., 2008a). Indeed, the Dartmouth COOP charts were designed with this purpose in mind (Nelson et al., 1996; de Azevedo-Marques and Zuardi, 2011) and evidence suggests that both patients and clinicians believe the use of the charts led to improved interaction, and better treatment. The use of such instruments may help to increase doctors' awareness of patients' problems, leading to more effective emotional and practical support (Detmar et al., 2002). While PROMs may provide useful information in the clinical interview, a systematic review of studies evaluating feedback of PROMs to health professionals found that the information was rarely passed on to patients (Luckett et al., 2009). Furthermore, it must be stressed that most PROMs were developed for use at the group, and not individual, level. Consequently, published indicators of their validity and reliability may not apply to individual scores. Lack of accuracy at the level of the individual may render interpretation of scores in this way meaningless (Donaldson, 2008).

Perhaps the most controversial use of health status measures is in the arena of cost containment and prioritization. Measures from which a single score can be derived are required for cost–utility studies, which seek to rank order treatments, or indeed patients. This figure, which represents the health state of the respondent, is weighted by values gained from the general population, which are intended to reflect societal views of any given health state. One of the most widely used of the 'utility measures' is the EuroQol EQ-5D (EuroQol Group, 1990). The EuroQol EQ-5D includes five questions covering mobility, self-care, usual activity, pain/discomfort, and anxiety/depression. Each question has three response categories: level 1—'no problems', level 2—'some problems', and level 3—'inability or extreme problems'. Overall health state can ostensibly be calculated from responses to these items. For example, the response set '11111' indicates no problems with any of the five areas, and subsequently perfect overall health. There are, in total, 243 possible health states (i.e. 3^5), and weighted values have been assigned to each of these on the basis of national and international surveys (van Agt et al., 1994). More recently, a version with five response options has been developed to increase the sensitivity and precision of the original instrument (Herdman et al., 2011), although as yet it has not been widely used. The data gained from the EQ-5D can be used to provide the 'quality' component in quality-adjusted life years (QALYs), which is an adjustment of life expectancy taking into account health status. It is then possible to determine the cost per QALY of treatments. Such information is used by the UK's National Institute for Health and Clinical Excellence to guide their recommendations on the cost-effectiveness of treatments.

Criteria for developing and assessing PROMs

Rating scales and questionnaires are not new to medicine, but traditionally such assessments were the product of clinical opinion, and, indeed, designed to be completed by physicians not patients. Many such instruments remain in use today, but the focus of PROMs is to place the patient at the centre of evaluation. PROMs should always be developed with patient input, for example, from in-depth interviews (Chapter 5) or focus groups (Chapter 6). Questions should reflect issues that are salient to patients, and be worded in a way that is meaningful to them. It is also important that the questionnaires comply with certain statistical and psychometric requirements, at the very least providing evidence of validity, reliability, and sensitivity to change.

Face validity refers to whether items on a questionnaire appear to be addressing the intended concept. This criterion is typically assessed by professional judgement. Content validity refers to whether the questions in an instrument cover all relevant domains or aspects of an intended topic or concept. In the *development* of PROMs patients are central to determining the content. They should be consulted at the item generation stage, and again when the draft measure has been constructed. Expert review, with clinicians or other relevant stakeholders, may also be undertaken to ensure nothing of great importance has been omitted. When *selecting* a questionnaire the importance of reading the content of a measure cannot be over-stressed. Simply basing choice of a measure on the titles of domains or published psychometric evidence is not sufficient. Many domain names, for instance, only give a broad indication of what is being measured; for example, 'social functioning' may refer to the quality of one's relationships with others, or the frequency of social contact.

Construct validity assesses the extent to which items are measuring an underlying construct, for example, 'social isolation'. It usually involves examining a whole pattern of correlations of the new construct with scores from other instruments that are presumed to be measuring related phenomena. When evaluating newly developed questionnaires it is usual practice for domains on the new measure to be compared with domains on a pre-existing, often generic, measure to establish convergent validity. The intention is not to seek perfect correlation, but rather similar trends in scores thereby supporting the measurement properties of the newer measure.

Criterion validity refers to the ability of an instrument to correspond with other measures held up as 'gold standards'. In practice, few studies can truly claim to have evaluated criterion validity as there are rarely gold standards for subjective phenomena. However, when a shorter form of a measure is being compared to the original longer version, the original long form can be viewed as the 'gold standard'. For example, the results of the physical and mental health summary scales from the 36-item SF-36 have been compared with results from the 12-item version of the questionnaire and have been found to be almost identical (Jenkinson et al., 1997).

Questionnaires must be reliable over time. Thus, they should produce the same, or very similar, results on two or more administrations to the same respondent, provided, of course, there is good reason to believe that the health status of the patient has not changed. Respondents could be asked if they have experienced any change since they initially completed the measure, and only those who claim to have experienced no change would contribute to the intraclass correlations. Internal consistency reliability can be calculated for items constituting a domain. This involves checking whether items in a scale are all measuring the same underlying construct reflected in the pattern of responses. Typically, internal consistency is measured using Cronbach's alpha statistic (Cronbach, 1951). Results below 0.6 are regarded as low, indicating that items in a scale are not all tapping the same underlying phenomena.

It is essential that evaluative instruments are able to detect change, and the level of this change is interpretable (Guyatt et al., 1987). This sensitivity or 'responsiveness' of an instrument is a very important criterion to consider when selecting measures to assess change. Questionnaire developers often publish data specifying 'minimally important differences' (MIDs), that is, the smallest change that can be detected on the measure that is meaningful to patients. The MID is the mean change in a score reported by respondents who indicate, in a follow-up study, that they had noticed some small change (Juniper et al., 1994). However, it should be borne in mind that estimates of responsiveness and minimal change vary across studies due to variability in populations, responses to treatments, and context. Therefore it has been suggested that several indices of minimal change are calculated, and for them to triangulate towards a range of values, in which confidence increases with replication (Revicki et al., 2006).

When selecting a measure for a given study it is important to consider the potential burden on respondents, evidence for alternative modes of administration, and ease of interpretation of data. The availability of validated translations may also need to be considered in, for example, international trials, as well as whether the mode of administration is acceptable. For example, recommendations have been drawn up for the evaluation of electronic computer administration of questionnaires originally designed for paper and pencil completion (Coons et al., 2009).

Tools have been developed to assist in the selection of PROMs—such as the EMPRO (Evaluating the Measurement of Patient Reported Outcomes) tool to assist in the choice of instruments against the earlier discussed criteria (Valderas et al., 2008b), and the COSMIN (COnsensus-based checklist for the Selection of health status Measurement INstruments) checklist to assess the quality of data provided in studies evaluating PROMs (Terwee et al., 2012).

New developments in measurement

A novel approach to assessment can be found in the form of individualized outcome measures. Individualized instruments take several forms, but a common theme is that individual respondents can nominate domains of concern to them and indicate the extent that such areas of life are compromised by illness. Examples of such instruments are the Schedule for the Evaluation of Individual Quality of Life (Direct Weighting version) (SEIQoL-DW) (Hickey et al., 1996) and the Patient Generated Index instrument (PGI) (Ruta et al., 1994). Such approaches to measurement certainly give a high priority to the individual's own view of what constitutes quality of life, but whether such scores can be viewed as measuring the same underlying phenomenon across individuals is controversial. Furthermore, the relatively complicated methods of eliciting responses have limited their uptake. They may, however, have high relevance for use in relation to medical consultations.

Typically PROMs have been designed for completion by pen and paper. Of course, questionnaires can potentially be completed by other means, such as face-to-face or telephone interviews, or electronically. Indeed, there is growing interest in computer-based PROMs, typically referred to as ePROs (electronic patient reported outcomes (Coons et al., 2009)). For the most part, the intention is to retain the original format and wording of the questionnaire on alternative platforms, although electronic platforms can permit for 'computerized adaptive testing' (CAT). CAT is predicated on the belief that not all items in a questionnaire may be relevant to all respondents. Thus, for example, someone who responds that they cannot walk 100 yards is unlikely to be able to walk a mile. Consequently, a CAT system will select subsequent questions on the basis of responses given by any given respondent (Chakravarty et al., 2007). Modern technology offers a range of exciting possibilities for rapid reporting and capture of patients' views about their health via PROMs.

Conclusions

The growth in PROMs, and their applications, is changing the way healthcare services are evaluated. The sheer number and variety of PROMs mean selection of instruments can be challenging, and many instruments do not provide clear guidance on interpretation of scores. For PROMs to be fully accepted, patients themselves must see some benefit from the data and consequently be willing to provide relevant information.

Looking forward, as PROMs become more widely accepted as an aspect of healthcare, a major challenge will be in raising patients' and the public's engagement, particularly if such data are to be used to contribute evidence of the quality of care. This will require asking new questions, for example, whether PROMs help patients monitor their health, communicate with health professionals, and choose treatments and services on the basis of PROMs from databases of other patients sharing their experiences. To date, PROMs have helped managers, researchers, and, more recently, healthcare providers in their roles. The future challenge is to make PROMs beneficial to patients and the public in making decisions that matter to them.

References

Chakravarty, E.F., Bjorner, J.B., and Fries, J.F. (2007). Improving patient reported outcomes using computerized adaptive testing and item response theory. *Journal of Rheumatology, 34*, 1426–31.

Coons, S.J., *et al.* (2009). Recommendations on evidence needed to support measure equivalence between electronic and paper-based patient reported outcome (PRO) measures: ISPOR ePRO good research practices task force report. *Value in Health, 12*, 419–29.

Cronbach, L.J. (1951). Coefficient alpha and the internal structure of tests. *Psychometrica, 16*, 297–334.

Darzi, A. (2008). *High quality care for all. NHS next stage review final report.* London: Department of Health.

Dawson, J., *et al.* (1996). Questionnaire on the perceptions of patients about total hip replacement. *Journal of Bone and Joint Surgery (Br), 78*, 185–90.

Dawson, J., *et al.* (2010). Routine use of patient reported outcome measures in healthcare settings. *British Medical Journal, 340*, 464–7.

de Azevedo-Marques, J.M. and Zuardi, A.W. (2011). COOP/WONCA charts as a screen for mental disorders in primary care. *Annals of Family Medicine, 9*, 359–65.

Detmar, S.B., *et al.* (2002). Health-related quality-of-life assessments and patient-physician communication: a randomized controlled trial. *Journal of the American Medical Association, 288*(23), 3027–34.

Donaldson, G. (2008). Patient-reported outcomes and the mandate of measurement. *Quality of Life Research, 17*, 1303–13.

EuroQol Group. (1990). EuroQol—a new facility for the measurement of health related quality of life. *Health Policy. 16*, 199–208.

Fitzpatrick, R., *et al.* (1992). Quality of life measures in health care. I: applications and issues in assessment. *British Medical Journal, 305*, 1074–7.

Fitzpatrick, R., *et al.* (1998). Evaluating patient based outcome measures for use in clinical trials. *Health Technology Assessment, 2*(14), 1–86.

Food and Drug Administration (2009). *Guidance for industry. Patient reported outcome measures: Use in medical product development to support labeling claims.* Silver Spring, MD: FDA.

Guyatt, G., Walter, S., and Norman, G. (1987). Measuring change over time: assessing the usefulness of evaluative instruments. *Journal of Chronic Diseases, 40*, 171–8.

Herdman, M., *et al.* (2011). Development and preliminary testing of the new five level EQ-5D (EQ-5D-5L). *Quality of Life Research, 20*, 1727–36.

Hickey, A.M., *et al.* (1996). A new short form quality of life measure (SEIQoL-DW): application in a cohort of individuals with HIV/AIDS. *British Medical Journal, 313*, 29–33.

Jenkinson, C., *et al.* (1997). A shorter form health survey: can the SF-12 replicate results from the SF-36 in longitudinal studies? *Journal of Public Health Medicine, 19*, 179–86.

Jenkinson, C., Fitzpatrick, R., and Peto, V. (2012). *PDQ-39 user manual* (3rd edn). Oxford: Health Services Research Unit.

Juniper, E., *et al.* (1994). Determining a minimally important change in a disease specific quality of life questionnaire. *Journal of Clinical Epidemiology, 47*, 81–7.

Lansky, D., Butler, J.B., and Waller, F.T. (1992). Using health status measures in the hospital setting: from acute care to 'outcomes management'. *Medical Care, 30*(Suppl. 5), MS57–MS73.

Luckett, T., Butow, P.N., and King, M.T. (2009). Improving patient outcomes through the routine use of patient-reported data in cancer clinics: future directions. *Psychooncology, 18*, 1129–38.

Nelson, E.C., *et al.* (1996). Dartmouth COOP functional assessment charts: brief measures for clinical practice. In: Spilker, B. (ed.) *Quality of life and pharmacoeconomics in clinical trials* (2nd edn), pp. 161–8. Philadelphia, PA: Lippincott-Raven.

Osaba, D. (2005). Health-related quality of life outcomes in clinical trials. In Fayers, P. and Hays, R. (eds) *Assessing quality of life in clinical trials* (2nd edn), pp. 259–74. Oxford: Oxford University Press.

Osaba, D., *et al.* (2000). Health-related quality of life in patients treated with temozolomide versus procarbazine for recurrent gliobastomamultiforme. *Journal of Clinical Oncology, 18*, 1481–91.

Revicki, D.A., *et al.* (2006). Responsiveness and minimal important differences for patient reported outcomes. *Health & Quality of Life Outcomes, 27*, 70.

Ruta, D.A., *et al.* (1994). A new approach to the measurement of quality of life. The Patient-Generated Index. *Medical Care, 32*, 1109–26.

Terwee, C.B., *et al.* (2012). Rating the methodological quality in systematic reviews of studies on measurement properties: a scoring system for the COSMIN checklist. *Quality of Life Research, 21*, 651–7.

Valderas, J.M., *et al.* (2008a). The impact of measuring patient-reported outcomes in clinical practice: a systematic review of the literature. *Quality of Life Research, 17*, 179–93.

Valderas J.M., *et al.* (2008b). Development of EMPRO: A tool for the standardised assessment of patient reported outcome measures. *Value in Health, 11*, 700–8.

Valderas, J.M., Fitzpatrick, R., and Roland, M. (2012). Using health status to measure NHS performance: another step into the dark for health reform in England. *BMJ Quality and Safety, 21*, 352–3.

van Agt, H.M.E., *et al.* (1994). Test-retest reliability of health state valuations collecting using the EuroQol questionnaire. *Social Science and Medicine, 39*, 1537–44.

Ware, J. (2007). *User's manual for the SF-36v2™ Health Survey* (2nd edn). Lincoln, RI: QualityMetric.

Williams, A., *et al.* (2010). Deep brain stimulation plus best medical therapy versus best medical therapy alone for advanced Parkinson's disease (PD SURG trial): a randomised, open label trial. *Lancet Neurology, 9*, 581–91.

Chapter 9

Patient experience surveys

Chris Graham and Penny Woods

Surveys are everywhere in academia, commerce , and public policy. Customer surveys, opinion polling, and social surveys, are increasingly widespread in modern life (e.g. Groves, 2011). Surveys measure social and personal preferences and experiences, and often this measurement is intended to support improvement in products or services.

Healthcare services are motivated to improve by a number of factors. Firstly, there is a moral imperative for providers to improve their services; commitment to excellence and continuous improvement are core elements of medical professionalism (Swick, 2000). Political interest and targets are also an influence, and in the 21st century these have increasingly focused on patients' experience (see Chapter 15). In many nations, providers also compete for patients, making improvement a business, as well as a healthcare, need. With the increasing recognition that patients' experiences represent a fundamental aspect of healthcare quality (Darzi, 2008), patient experience surveys are key to generating information for providers, commissioners, regulators, and users of healthcare services.

Here, we outline the range of survey approaches available to measure patient experience, and address their characteristics and the design choices that must underpin them. First, though, we briefly review the history of patient experience surveys.

History

Patient *experience* surveys have their roots in patient *satisfaction* surveys, although there are marked differences in the underlying approach. Surveys of patient satisfaction first emerged in the 1950s (Abdellah and Levine, 1957), with research typically focusing on the quality of personal interactions (Korsch et al., 1968). The measurement of patient satisfaction developed greater prominence in the 1980s. In England, the National Health Service (NHS) Management Inquiry (1983, p. 1393) recommended that the NHS should seek to 'ascertain how well the service is being delivered...by obtaining the experiences and perceptions of patients', notably via market research. Similarly, patient satisfaction was advocated as an indicator of quality in the USA (Cleary and McNeil, 1988).

Contemporaneously, some reviewers began to question the conceptual validity of patient satisfaction. 'Satisfaction' is too simplistic and vaguely defined to provide adequate measures of the experiences and perceptions of patients (Williams, 1994). Moreover, data on satisfaction has limited utility for service improvement: knowing that a patient was dissatisfied suggests a *need* for improvement, but provides no information on *why* that patient was dissatisfied or how this could be addressed. Consequently research into patient feedback began to focus on reports of experiences rather than satisfaction (Cleary, 1998). With a growing global trend towards patient-centred care (see Chapter 2), patient experience surveys have since been widely adopted.

The principles of patient experience surveys have changed little since the late 1990s. In contrast to satisfaction surveys, which seek to evaluate some overall sense of contentment with services, patient experience surveys ask people to report on what happened to them during their care. Whilst the most important aspects of care vary between individuals and groups, patient experience approaches assume that specific characteristics of care are of value to most patients. Examining whether these characteristics are present in people's reports of care therefore allows for relatively objective evaluation of whether care was provided in a way consistent with good experiences. Particularly, questions focus on specific, reportable events reflecting areas shown to be important: for example, *reporting* whether things did or did not happen rather than *rating* satisfaction. This minimizes the need for respondents to make evaluations and allows individual reports to be framed within patient experience more broadly.

A wide range of patient experience surveys are used. In England there are regular national surveys of people accessing general practitioners (GPs), hospitals, and mental health services. Many healthcare providers undertake their own surveys, often using technology to record feedback in 'near real-time' (Robert et al., 2011). CAHPS (Consumer Assessment of Healthcare Providers and Systems) surveys are widely used in the USA, whilst many other countries—including Japan, Australia, and Switzerland—operate national patient surveys. The importance ascribed to these surveys has grown. In England, for example, patient survey results are linked to payments for hospitals and GPs and contribute to clinicians' revalidation from December 2012 (General Medical Council, 2012).

Survey development

Most quantitative surveys rely predominantly on closed questions, perhaps supplemented with a few open-ended questions or a comments box. This ensures data collected will be consistently structured, but also imposes an important limitation: the survey will, by and large, only provide feedback on things that are explicitly asked about. Getting the content right is therefore vital, and it is important to take patients' perspectives into account. This means not only picking topics that are important to patients but also ensuring that the questions themselves are appropriate and understandable.

There is long-standing recognition that qualitative methods should inform questionnaire design. For example, Lazarsfeld (1944) notes the 'invaluable' role of open-ended depth interviews (Chapter 5) in identifying topics and terms for survey design. Focus groups (Chapter 6) can also be used (Wolff et al., 1993), both to inform the choice of questions and to help to refine wording and response categories.

Mixed-method approaches to survey development are particularly relevant in healthcare where surveys aspire to measure what matters to patients. England's NHS Patient Survey Programme, for example, uses focus groups to explore the particular view of NHS users when adapting questionnaires originally developed for other health services (Reeves et al., 2002).

Once a draft questionnaire has been developed, some form of validation is usually appropriate. Questions drafted by researchers may possess good face validity—they may *appear* comprehensible and salient—but not make sense to patients. Good item design is essential: otherwise results may be unusable or, worse, actively misleading. Some misleading items may not even be identified during a pilot phase of the survey: that people respond to questions does not necessarily mean that they have understood them as intended.

Cognitive interviewing is a particularly powerful, usually iterative, approach to testing and validating survey instruments (Willis, 2005; Beatty and Willis, 2007). Essentially, this involves asking people observed by a researcher to complete a questionnaire and 'think aloud' as they do so. Researchers may also 'probe' by asking people for their interpretation of particular terms or questions. This illuminates the cognitive process of responding, and allows researchers to identify potential issues with how people comprehend questions, retrieve information from memory, evaluate questions, and indicate their response (Tourangeau, 1984). The purpose of the survey should be taken into account, and questions designed accordingly.

Surveys focused on driving improvements should identify actionable information on where this is scope for improvement. Contrastingly, surveys for performance assessment must produce data suitable for facilitating comparisons. Questions should be simple, direct, and unambiguous. They should also avoid medical or clinical jargon and give appropriate response options (see Figure 9.1 for an illustration of an inappropriate question and how this

Hospital patients are often given medications to take at home after discharge. Hospital staff must ensure people are given adequate information about their medicines. **Qa** and **Qb** below both seek to address this.

Qa. Were you told what your medicines were for and how to take them?	**Qb.** Were you told **how** to take your medication in a way you could understand?
☐ Yes ☐ No	☐ Yes, definitely ☐ Yes, to some extent ☐ No ☐ I did not need to be told how to take my medication

Qa is flawed whilst **Qb** represents an improved, good practice alternative. Key issues are:

- **Qa** is 'double-barrelled': it asks whether patients were told both about the *purpose* and *usage* of medicines. It is better to ask the questions separately.

- A simple yes/no does not allow for the possibility of receiving some information but not enough. Adding an intermediary 'yes, to some extent' option addresses this.

- **Qa** does not give people an opportunity to say if the question is not relevant to them. Adding an "I did not need to be told" option in the second version takes better account of situations where information is genuinely not needed and avoids the seemingly negative option of 'no' being selected instead.

- In spite of the revisions, the item would be confusing for people who were not given any medications to take away. This could be addressed with a 'screening' question asking whether people were given any medications.

Qb. in figure 9.1 is reproduced from the NHS adult inpatient survey and is copyright of the Care Quality Commission (CQC). This question is reproduced with permission from CQC.

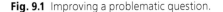

Fig. 9.1 Improving a problematic question.

could be improved). Sensitivity to the healthcare context is also needed since items used successfully in other sectors may not translate well to patient surveys. For example, the 'Net Promoter Score' (Reichheld, 2003) is widely used in commercial settings but has been shown to be inappropriate for use in NHS national patient surveys (Graham and MacCormick, 2012).

Finally, it should be noted that it is rarely necessary to develop a questionnaire from scratch—there are many tested and validated measures. Designing new questions can be counter-productive, frustrating comparisons between services and across time. For example, Robert et al. (2011) examined electronic surveys used by many NHS providers and found 18 different versions of a question asking patients about whether they were treated with respect and dignity. These variations made it impossible to directly compare results between providers.

Sampling

Typically, quantitative patient surveys use probability samples, where eligible patients on a sampling frame each have a known probability of selection. Probability samples rely on known statistical properties to allow results to be generalized to the wider population. A properly drawn sample can produce reliable estimates about the experiences of much larger groups. Even relatively small probability samples are likely to produce more representative results than larger surveys that do not use statistical sampling. Larger samples add little precision to estimates about an overall population: for example, a random sample of fewer than 1,100 people will produce estimates with a maximum margin of error of ±3%, but to reduce this to ±1% requires almost nine times as large a sample.

Simple random samples and systematic samples are the most straightforward and commonly used. More complex approaches involve sampling with non-equal probability of selection. Typically, non-equal probability sampling strategies aim to ensure that key demographic groups are properly represented in the sample. Stratification of the sample frame may be used to 'boost' the response from smaller groups by giving them a disproportionately high likelihood of selection. This is particularly valuable for addressing health inequalities as adequate data can be collected from minority groups without implications for overall sample size. Statistical adjustment such as design weighting is normally then required to produce population-level estimates from the survey data.

Probability sampling approaches will not always be feasible: in such cases a non-probability or 'convenience' sample may be used. This will not allow results to be generalized back to a wider population or compared across organizations, but it need not prevent the survey data being used for service improvement, especially if a reasonable volume of data is collected and the limitations of the data are noted. Again, the methodological approach needs to take into account the reasons for doing the survey.

The proportion of people in the sample completing the survey (known as the response rate) is always important. It is not the *number* of respondents so much as their representativeness that is important—and the two will not always be correlated. Whilst high response rates are always desirable it is important to investigate whether some groups are more likely to respond than others: this can lead to non-response bias.

Mode of administration

Surveys can be administered via a variety of 'modes', from face-to-face interviews to online surveys. Different survey modes have very different practical and theoretical characteristics, and there is no one 'best' method to use. Each approach has its own strengths and weaknesses, and the choice of survey mode for a project usually involves a cost–benefit trade off. For example, interview-administered modes will typically yield higher response rates than self-administered surveys—albeit at considerably higher costs. Postal surveys remain popular because they can be sent to large numbers of patients to collect high volumes of robust, standardized data at acceptable cost—but they also take a relatively long time to produce results. A fuller discussion of different modes of administration can be found in Graham (2007).

Results obtained from any survey are inextricably linked to its design, and surveys using different modes may obtain different results even when asking identical questions. This is due to how the items are presented and how respondents interact with questions and response scales. Different sources of bias may come into play in different settings. For example, acquiescence and socially desirable responding are more common in interview-administered survey methods (Schuman and Presser, 1981; Groves, 1989)—particularly when questions relate to sensitive topics (Tourangeau and Smith, 1996). These 'mode effects' are particularly important in surveys that employ 'mixed-mode' methodologies, using more than one approach to collect data from different people (De Leeuw, 2005).

Another important distinction is between retrospective surveys conducted after a patient has completed a healthcare episode and 'near real-time' surveys conducted during an episode. Whilst there is a limited research base around near real-time approaches, which have only recently come into vogue, patients are more likely to give positive responses about care they are currently receiving. For example, a Healthcare Commission (2005a) report compared the results of a postal survey with another survey using bedside televisions in hospitals. The surveys involved similar groups of patients and asked near identical questions. Results differed markedly: for example, 46% of postal survey and 58% of bedside respondents said bathrooms were 'very clean'. Similar findings are frequently observed in routine hospital surveys, lending support to the idea that experience is likely to be more positively reported whilst care is ongoing. We are not aware of published trials systematically evaluating the effect of the identity of interviewers in in-hospital surveys, but it is reasonable to expect more acquiescence and socially desirable responding if a survey is administered by staff.

Analysis and reporting

Appropriate analysis and reporting is essential to maximizing value from patient experience surveys and should, ideally, be planned at the earliest stages.

Several issues should be considered when interpreting survey data—especially when comparing results between sites or over time. Changes or differences in the demographic characteristics of respondents can influence results, because some groups are likely to respond differently to others in most surveys. Older people tend to respond more positively to healthcare surveys (Bowling, 2002), as do men (Sizmur, 2011). By contrast, patients from black and minority ethnic (BME) groups are typically less positive about their experiences (Department of Health, 2009). Specific differences may also be encountered in particular healthcare settings: in the case of hospital inpatients, those admitted in an emergency tend to be less positive than those with a planned admission (Healthcare Commission, 2005b, 2006). Groups with different response characteristics also often differ in overall response rates, so care is needed to ensure results are not biased by disproportionate nonresponse from certain groups. For example, people from BME groups and younger people are typically not only less positive in their responses but also considerably less likely to respond at all (Sheldon et al., 2007).

This can influence comparisons when there are differences in patient populations. Consider a hospital with a very young population: we might expect it to have comparatively poor survey results because younger patients typically report poorer experiences. This can be addressed in several ways—either by using stratified sampling, limiting comparisons to those within certain demographic groups, or by statistically 'weighting' the data to standardize for these differences. Weighting involves selectively modifying the extent to which each respondent's answers contribute to the survey results: this can be used to balance demographic differences and create a 'level playing field' for comparisons. Although weighting is useful for performance management or assessment across organizations, it can be less helpful for quality improvement purposes. Typically weights reflect external populations—for example, the case mix of an 'average hospital'—but this can remove or obfuscate issues related to local populations. Changing one's case mix is rarely an option for staff looking to improve services: rather, the focus should be on understanding and improving the experiences of local populations, for which unweighted, locally representative data may be more appropriate.

Confidentiality is another important issue when analysing survey results. Typically, patient surveys are confidential or anonymous—but care must still be taken to ensure that respondents are not inadvertently identified. To minimize this risk, it is common practice to suppress results based on groups of fewer than 20 or 30 respondents: this also avoids untoward focus on unreliable data. Discretion should also be used if presenting verbatim comments, which may require a different analytic approach (e.g. Garcia et al., 2004).

Service improvement

Most patient surveys include 'service improvement' as an aim: using the data to identify and remedy shortcomings in existing services. This aspect of a patient survey is, we believe, the most important of all—but it is all too easy to neglect.

In England, almost all major public sector healthcare providers receive patient feedback via surveys at least annually. Yet this information is not always fully utilized for quality improvement—and the reasons for this highlight some of the factors that should be in place to support meaningful quality improvement.

Firstly, survey results are not always given due attention at a senior level. Leadership and commitment has been described as 'the single most important factor contributing to patient-centred care' (Shaller, 2007, p. 13). Despite this, a recent review of minutes and agendas from NHS hospital trusts found that in 95% of cases where boards discussed patient experience 'the minuted action point...[was] to note the report and take no further action' (Robert et al., 2011, p. 16).

Secondly, getting the right data at the right time is important. One of the most commonly reported barriers to using patient survey data is that it is not 'granular' enough—the data is not specific to individual wards or teams—or that it is not updated frequently enough to provide regular measures of changes (Reeves and Seccombe, 2008). These issues should be taken into account when planning surveys. If, for example, the aim of a survey is to identify the best wards in a hospital and share their good practice with others, then the sample size for the survey should be sufficiently large to provide reliable data for each ward (see Figure 9.2).

Those involved in quality improvement also value comparative data from similar providers to contextualize results, provide benchmarks, and make comparisons over time (Reeves and Seccombe, 2008). Longitudinal data is particularly valued and can become part of a cycle of improvement and measurement. Delivering both robust inter-organization comparisons and frequent longitudinal data can be challenging, though, because of the time required to produce standardized, large-scale datasets. Triangulating information from different sources can be useful—such as by using near real-time feedback for regular updates between less frequent 'milestone' surveys. Novel approaches to triangulation may include data from very different sources, for example, linking national survey results to clinical audit data (Howell et al., 2007) or ratings submitted online (Greaves et al., 2012).

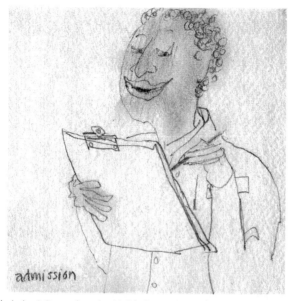

Fig. 9.2 'Admission'. Reproduced with kind permission from Nick Wadley, *Man + Doctor*, Dalkey Archive Press, London, UK, Copyright© 2012 Nick Wadley.

These points demonstrate the importance of tailoring survey design to planned use. Surveys intended to inform quality improvement require senior level support. Similarly, thought should be given to both the frequency and the level at which surveys will report: feedback given regularly and at the level of individual units or even clinicians is more likely to be 'owned' by the relevant staff. Frequent and detailed reporting is costly and will not always be necessary if the aim of a large survey is to compare organizations or to report population level data.

Conclusions

In this chapter we have addressed some of the key characteristics and considerations around patient experience surveys. This is intended to give a sense of the range of issues that should be addressed in the planning and implementation of a good survey. To conclude, it is worth reviewing the strengths and weaknesses of surveys.

Firstly, surveys are highly structured. This makes them suitable for collecting large volumes of comparable quantitative data. This, along with good sampling methods, allows survey data to be generalized beyond the population of respondents. It also enables statistical analyses that would not be possible with less structured data. However, the process is inevitably somewhat top-down. Reliance on closed-questions means that surveys largely tell us only what we ask about, leaving limited scope for unexpected feedback to 'bubble up' from respondents. This can be partially addressed by inviting 'any other comments': however, qualitative data received from this can be time-consuming to analyse, especially in larger surveys, and can be difficult to integrate into other survey results (Garcia et al., 2004).

There are also practical advantages to surveys. Because they rely on standardized tools and methods, surveys are highly scalable: once questionnaires and methodologies are developed they can be implemented widely and repeated easily. This is especially true of postal and online surveys but less so in the more labour intensive interviewer-administered methods. Scalable, repeatable methods are extremely useful because they can easily be extended beyond the initial population of interest or repeated to generate comparative or longitudinal data. However, the more scalable methods can also be more time-consuming. Postal surveys in particular need to be run for an appropriate length of time for responses to accumulate, and reminder letters will be needed to help with this (e.g. Dillman et al., 2009).

Ensuring an appropriate sample size can be a challenge. Whilst relatively small samples can be successfully used to produce reliable estimates for populations, sample size requirements increase when data is to be compared between a number of groups, wards, or organizations. This can make traditional survey methods costly, so it is often appropriate to consider how the rigorously collected data from cross-sectional surveys can be supplemented with other work. Using qualitative methods to follow up survey results can be particularly helpful where results indicate a problem and more detail is needed. For example, a survey might show that patients feel that they are given too little information about their treatment; semi-structured interviews could establish exactly what kind of information was missing and how this could be addressed.

The issues considered in this chapter all emphasize the importance of ensuring that survey methods are appropriate to their intended use. Giving due regard to decisions around survey methodology and content will help to ensure that results are useful and actionable. Involving patients in the design of surveys is vital, as this can ensure that surveys measure what matters to patients as well as demonstrating the validity of question content. Similarly, taking account of the views of people using surveys for service improvement can help to make results as useful as possible. This is likely to include thinking about how to balance granularity and cost, timeliness, and rigour. When conducted well, though, there is little doubt that surveys of patients can provide important data for organizations to measure and to improve their performance, and surveys are likely to remain a key tool for measuring and understanding patients' experiences.

Further reading

Dillman, D.A., Smyth, J.D., and Christian, L.M. (2009). *Internet, mail, and mixed-mode surveys: The tailored design method.* New York, NY: Wiley.

Lohr, S. (2010). *Sampling: design and analysis* (2nd edn). Pacific Grove, CA: Brooks/Cole.

See <http://www.nhssurveys.org> for further information on the NHS Patient Survey Programme in England. The site provides a range of resources including tested questionnaires for local use.

References

Abdellah, F.G., and Levine, E. (1957). Developing a measure of patient and personnel satisfaction with nursing care. *Nursing Research, 5*(3), 100–8.

Beatty, P.C. and Willis, G.B. (2007). Research synthesis: the practice of cognitive interviewing. *Public Opinion Quarterly, 71*(2), 287–311.

Bowling, A. (2002). An 'inverse satisfaction law'? Why don't older patients criticise health services? *Journal of Epidemiology and Community Health, 56*(7), 482.

Cleary, P.D. and McNeil, B.J. (1988). Patient satisfaction as an indicator of quality care. *Inquiry, 25*(1), 25–36.

Cleary, P.D. (1998). Satisfaction may not suffice! A commentary on 'a patient's perspective'. *International Journal of Technology Assessment in Health Care, 14*(1), 35–7.

Darzi, A. (2008). Quality and the NHS next stage review. *Lancet, 371*(9624), 1563.

De Leeuw, E.D. (2005). To mix or not to mix data collection modes in surveys. *Journal of Official Statistics, 21*(5), 233–55.

Department of Health. (2009). *Report on the self reported experience of patients from black and minority ethnic groups.* London: Department of Health. Available at: <http://www.dh.gov.uk/prod_consum_dh/groups/dh_digitalassets/documents/digitalasset/dh_100471.pdf> (accessed 5 March 2012).

Dillman, D.A., Smyth, J.D., and Christian, L.M. (2009). *Internet, mail, and mixed-mode surveys: The tailored design method.* New York, NY: Wiley.

Garcia, J., Evans, J., and Reshaw, M. (2004). 'Is there anything else you would like to tell us'—methodological issues in the use of free-text comments from postal surveys. *Quality & Quantity, 38*(2), 113–25.

General Medical Council. (2012). *Revalidation | Getting involved.* [Online] Available at: <http://www.gmc-uk.org/doctors/revalidation/12397.asp> (accessed 8 August 2012).

Graham, C. (2007). *Mixed mode surveys: A review for the NHS acute patient survey programme.* Oxford: Picker Institute Europe.

Graham, C. and MacCormick, S. (2012). *Overarching questions for patient surveys: development report for the Care Quality Commission (CQC).* Oxford: Picker Institute Europe. Available at: <http://www.nhssurveys.org/survey/1186> (accessed 21 June 2012).

Greaves, F., *et al.* (2012). Associations between internet-based patient ratings and conventional surveys of patient experience in the English NHS: an observational study. *BMJ Quality and Safety, 21*, 600–5.

Groves, R.M. (1989). *Survey errors and survey costs*. New York, NY: Wiley.

Groves, R.M. (2011). Three eras of survey research. *Public Opinion Quarterly*, *75*(5), 861–71.

Healthcare Commission. (2005a). *A snapshot of hospital cleanliness in England*. London: Healthcare Commission.

Healthcare Commission. (2005b). *Variations in the experiences of patients in England: Analysis of the Healthcare Commission's 2003/2004 national surveys of patients*. London: Healthcare Commission. Available at: <http://archive.cqc.org.uk/_db/_documents/04021207.pdf> (accessed 5 March 2012).

Healthcare Commission. (2006). *Variations in the experiences of patients in England: Analysis of the Healthcare Commission's 2004/2005 national surveys of patients*. London: Healthcare Commission.

Howell, E., *et al.* (2007). Comparison of patients' assessments of the quality of stroke care with audit findings. *Quality and Safety in Health Care*, *16*(6), 450–5.

Korsch, B.M., Gozzi, E.K., and Francis, V. (1968). Gaps in doctor-patient communication. 1. Doctor-patient interaction and patient satisfaction. *Pediatrics*, *42*(5), 855–71.

Lazarsfeld, P.J. (1944). The controversy over detailed interviews—an offer for negotiation. *Public Opinion Quarterly*, *8*(1), 38–60.

NHS Management Inquiry. (1983). Small, central management board recommended. *British Medical Journal (Clinical Research Edition)*, *287*(6402), 1391–4.

Reeves, R., *et al.* (2002). *Development and pilot testing of questionnaires for use in the acute NHS trust inpatient survey programme*. Oxford: Picker Institute Europe.

Reeves, R. and Seccombe, I. (2008). Do patient surveys work? The influence of a national survey programme on local quality-improvement initiatives. *Quality and Safety in Health Care*, *17*(6), 437–41.

Reichheld, F.F. (2003). The one number you need to grow. *Harvard Business Review*, *81*(12), 46–55.

Robert, G., *et al.* (2011). *'What matters to patients?': Developing the evidence base for measuring and improving patient experience*. London: NHS Institute for Innovation and Improvement. Available at: <http://www.institute.nhs.uk/images/Patient_Experience/Final%20Project%20Report%20pdf%20doc%20january%202012.pdf> (accessed 26 April 2012).

Schuman, H. and Presser, S. (1981). *Questions and answers in attitude surveys*. New York, NY: Academic Press.

Shaller, D. (2007). *Patient-centered care: What does it take? Report for the Picker Institute and the Commonwealth Fund*. New York, NY: The Commonwealth Fund. Available at: <http://www.commonwealthfund.org/~/media/Files/Publications/Fund%20Report/2007/Oct/Patient%20Centered%20Care%20%20What%20Does%20It%20Take/Shaller_patient%20centeredcarewhatdoesittake_1067%20pdf.pdf>.

Sheldon, H., *et al.* (2007). *Increasing response rates amongst black and minority ethnic and 'seldom heard' groups*. Oxford: Picker Institute. Available at: <http://www.nhssurveys.org/Filestore/documents/Increasing_response_rates_literature_review.pdf> (accessed 2 August 2012).

Sizmur, S. (2011). *Multilevel analysis of inpatient experience*. Oxford: Picker Institute Europe. Available at: <http://pickereurope.org/assets/content/pdf/Survey_data_analyses/

Multilevel_analysis_of_inpatient_Experience_March_2011.pdf> (accessed 6 March 2012).

Swick, H.M. (2000). Toward a normative definition of medical professionalism. *Academic Medicine*, 75(6), 612–16.

Tourangeau, R. (1984). Cognitive sciences and survey methods. In Jabine, T., *et al.* (eds) *Cognitive aspects of survey methodology: Building a bridge between disciplines*, pp. 73–100. Washington, DC: National Academy Press.

Tourangeau, R. and Smith, T.W. (1996). Asking sensitive questions: the impact of data collection mode, question format, and question context. *Public Opinion Quarterly, 60*, 275–304.

Williams, B. (1994). Patient satisfaction: a valid concept? *Social Science & Medicine, 38*(4), 509–16.

Willis, G.B. (2005). *Cognitive interviewing: A tool for improving questionnaire design.* London: Sage.

Wolff, B., Knodel, J., and Sittitrai, W. (1993). Focus groups and surveys as complementary research methods. In Morgan, D. (ed.) *Successful focus groups: Advancing the state of the art*, pp. 118–36. London: Sage.

Chapter 10

Using the Internet as a source of information about patients' experiences

Fadhila Mazanderani and John Powell

Introduction

The Internet has become a major repository of health information. While a great deal of the information available online is supplied by healthcare providers, pharmaceutical companies, and other organizations from the public, private, and charity sectors, there is an ever growing body of content generated by people living with or caring for someone with a health condition. Such user-generated content includes personal stories and testimonials found in blogs and personal websites, discussions based on individual experience found in forums and chat-rooms, feedback captured by patient opinion and ratings websites, and an increasing number of health-related exchanges on social media platforms. As the web has evolved from a largely text-based to a multimedia environment, and users are increasingly able to connect from anywhere at broadband speeds, often using mobile devices, this user-generated content has grown to encompass photographs, audio, and video accounts of personal experience.

This chapter focuses on how user-generated experiential information on the Internet can be used as a resource for exploring patients' experiences. This type of content has been referred to as 'naturally occurring' and 'unsolicited' (Robinson, 2001; O'Brien and Clark, 2012), however, we avoid using these terms as researchers may choose to directly intervene in the online environments that they study (e.g. informing forum users that they are observing it) and information that has been 'solicited' (e.g. by a charitable organization as part of an awareness campaign) can also be a valuable source of data.

How to study online representations of patients' experiences

Initially the Internet was conceptualized as a 'virtual' or 'cyber' space, removed from and in contrast to the 'real' or 'physical' space people inhabit in their day-to-day lives. This resulted in an upsurge of contrasting cyber utopian and cyber dystopian perspectives. Overtime, aided by contextually sensitive approaches and the use of a variety of social science methods— interviews, surveys, ethnographies, content analysis (Hine, 2005)—there has been a shift towards conceptualizing the Internet as embedded within particular cultures and contexts of use (for an overview see Woolgar (2002)). This has been mirrored in studies focused specifically on patients' experiences online where there has been a shift from a reductionist concern with whether sharing experiences online is 'good' or 'bad' for people's health, towards nuanced analyses of the practices, representations, and implications of online experiential information sharing (Ziebland and Wyke, 2012)

As technologies change so too do the type of data available, and many websites and patient organizations have added to their online repertoire through the inclusion of forums, social networking sites (e.g. Facebook), micro blogging (e.g. Twitter), and video content (e.g. YouTube). Methods for studying these technologies are still in their formative stages and in addition to capturing (either manually or through automated scripts and technologies) the content contained in this media and analysing it, there is increased methodological (and often technological) innovation in this area. This opens up new opportunities for researchers interested in studying experiences of health and illness on and through the Internet. Yet, at the same time, it requires the development of new skills and increased sensitivity to the particular ethical norms and expectations of online environments.

Many of the research methods covered elsewhere in the book have been adapted and applied in online contexts. For example, in Chapter 3 Joseph Calabrese discusses ethnographic methods, observational studies of interpersonal interaction is considered by Fiona Stevenson in Chapter 4, and the analysis of narratives and patient stories are covered by Sue Ziebland and Trisha Greenhalgh in Chapters 5 and 6 respectively. We do not, therefore, cover these here. Instead we focus on how various versions of what can be considered 'content' analysis have been used as a means of collecting and analysing the vast array of health-related experiential information on the Internet.

Content analysis has been defined as the 'systematic reading of a body of texts, images, and symbolic matter' (Krippendorff, 2004, p. 3). Originating from studies of print media, it includes a range of quantitative and qualitative approaches that have been adapted and used in relation to the Internet. What we broadly refer to as content analysis includes many distinct methods and approaches. For example, thematic and narratives analyses (e.g. of HIV/AIDS activist websites (Gillett, 2003) and pro-anorexia forums (Fox et al. 2005)); conversation analysis, where detailed attention is paid to styles of speech, language use, and interaction (e.g. on a diabetes forum (Armstrong et al., 2012)); corpus linguistic and keywords analysis, where particular word and other linguistic occurrences are quantified and analysed (e.g. in relation to representations of cancer (Seale et al., 2006) and sexual health (Harvey et al., 2007)); and, more recently, the use of 'digital methods', where the very 'objects' of the Internet (hyperlinks, hash tags, search engines etc.), are used to study broader phenomenon, such as predict flu outbreaks (Rogers, 2010).

When studying online representations of patients' experiences, researchers have to tackle many of the same questions dealt with in more traditional research contexts. The methodological approach adopted needs to be driven by the research question not by the convenience of the data and careful consideration should be given to the medium and context under investigation. The specifics of your research design will depend on your disciplinary repertoire and research interests rather than on any generic guidelines, and may need to be adapted over time. Whichever approach is chosen, it will be helpful to undertake a scoping exercise, spending time observing and familiarizing yourself with the environment you intend to study, in order to better understand the potential data that is out there, how to best study it, and the challenges that might arise as the research progresses.

It is important to remember that people who choose to share their experiences online are not necessarily representative of the general population, and this needs to be recognized in relation to any claims you make in terms of generalizability and representativeness. Research consistently shows that Internet users tend to be younger, more educated, and from a higher income bracket than non-Internet users. The reduced cost and increased availability of broadband connections, and the growth of a younger generation of digital natives, is lessening this divide, but inequalities do still persist and need to be considered by researchers seeking to sample experiential information from online sources. In the next section, drawing on examples from existing research, we outline some key approaches, strengths, and insights that the analysis of online representations of patients' experiences can contribute to our understanding of people's experiences of health and illness.

Why study online representations of patients' experiences?

One of the most obvious ways in which the Internet can contribute to the study of patients' experiences is as a rich source of data that can replace and/or supplement other data sources. For example, Adair et al. (2006) used Internet-based first-person narratives to supplement qualitative material derived from other sources in the development of a quality-of-life instrument for eating disorders. They concluded that the Internet was an efficient, inexpensive, and productive source of data, and that the online narratives included some sensitive topics (later validated in focus groups) not obtained through their interview work.

Online, researchers can access a large, international, and diverse collection of patient stories and interactions that can facilitate research into many health-related topics, including those focused on rare conditions and hard-to-reach groups. Moreover, Internet technologies provide opportunities for studying personal accounts and interactions over time and in various formats. For example, in the paper by Armstrong et al. (2012), sequential posts in a diabetes forum were analysed to understand how issues of identity and authority become established over time. As technology adoption accelerates and mobile devices, such as smartphones combined with social media platforms, facilitate an 'always on' culture where personal experience is recorded and shared instantly, different technologies and digital methods enable the contemporaneous recording of experiential accounts. In contrast to this 'real-time' capture of data, the archival nature of the Internet provides opportunities for historical analysis of experiences of health and illness (e.g. through tools such as the Wayback machine at <http://www.archive.org>).

Furthermore, online content has played an important role in enabling researchers to examine the changing dynamics of the patient experience in contemporary healthcare more generally—often in relation to changes enabled in part by the use of Internet technologies. Activist websites, social media sites, and patient forums, have contributed to research on patient activism and health social movements. For example, Hobson-West (2007) used Internet postings as one of multiple sources of data in an analysis of the discourses of risk and trust produced by groups critical of vaccinations in the UK. Such an analysis provides insight into the dynamics of resistance to biomedical authority and healthcare policies, such as childhood measles, mumps, and rubella (MMR) vaccination (Skea et al., 2008).

An area of great interest to policymakers and healthcare providers is the recent trend in which patients use the Internet to share their opinions of and rate services (e.g. <http://www.patientopinion.org.uk>). A UK study by Greaves et al. (2012) examined the quality ratings provided by National Health Service (NHS) patients on their experiences of care posted on the NHS Choices website (<http://www.nhs.uk>) and correlated these with non-experiential measures of hospital performance. While the relationship was not clear cut, they found that overall patients' ratings of their experience of hospital care tallied with other measures of the hospital's performance, including mortality. Thus, as healthcare providers seek to drive quality improvement and increase transparency, online rating and reputational systems are emerging as tools for helping them do so through capturing patients' experiences of services.

One criticism frequently leveraged against research on patients' experiences is that too little attention is paid to the issue of how these experiences, be they articulated in stories, brief quotes, images, or numbers, are constructed. When we speak about representations of peoples' experiences of health and illness on the Internet, it is important to note that these representations should not be treated as depicting some reality 'out there', but as emerging through particular socially and technically mediated practices. Just as data collected through interviews and other methods are constructed in particular ways and for particular reasons, so too are experiences shared online and it is important that the researcher takes these different factors and contingencies into consideration (for a comparison between information generated through interviews and forums see Seale et al. (2010)).

People present themselves differently in different settings and it may be difficult, if not impossible, to verify the authenticity of an experience posted online or the (true) identity of the poster. And while this should definitely be taken into consideration in any analysis, this apparent difficulty provides many opportunities for researching issues relating to the construction, mediation, and communication of illness experiences. Forums, in particular, have been used as a rich source of data for understanding health-related communication and identity formation. For example, Horne and Wiggins (2009) analysed the messages posted in two suicide forums over a one-month period. Here, rather than simply categorizing forum posts as belonging to people experiencing suicidal thoughts, they examined how users established themselves as authentically suicidal.

Although health-related forums differ in many ways, they share common features and are usually based on a thematically organized bulletin board type service where users can browse the discussion board, post questions, and receive answers. While forums often contain private messaging services and can restrict access in various ways, they still provide a great deal of searchable data (e.g. based on topic, data, poster, etc.) that was simply not available before the Internet. In addition to enabling the analysis of self-presentation and identify formation, forums have been extensively studied in relation to how social and emotional support are performed through experiential information sharing (e.g. in the context of breast cancer (Orgad, 2006) and HIV/ADS (Bar-Lev, 2008)). As social media platforms such as Facebook and YouTube are increasingly used as a means of documenting and sharing experiences, it seems likely that they too shall be researched more extensively in relation to illness experiences.

Ethical considerations of researching patients' experiences online

While it might seem incredibly easy and convenient to analyse information on the Internet, it is important to ensure that this material is researched in an ethically appropriate manner. Different disciplines often have specific ethical guidelines for conducting online research (e.g. the British Psychological Association) and the Association of Internet Researchers guidelines cover many of the issues touched upon very briefly here (Ess, 2002).

A key factor to consider when negotiating the ethics of researching experiences that patients have posted online is the nature of the analysis you are conducting. Quantitative analyses that do not rely on extensive quotes and work with large corpuses of information will typically be easier to anonymize. However, when presenting qualitative research, and particularly discourse analysis, it is usually necessary to include large pieces of verbatim text. Even when anonymized, quotations can be pasted into a search engine and become potentially identifiable in their original setting, perhaps with attribution. In cases like this, difficult decisions will have to be made about what to include that will need to be assessed on a case-by-case basis and precautions, such as only directly quoting from publically available sources and not revealing the name of websites, may need to be taken.

One of the key dimensions to be considered when choosing what material to analyse and quote is the relative public or private nature of the environment being analysed. Drawing a strict distinction between whether online information is 'private' or 'public' will usually not be possible, but in some cases the information may be considered more straightforwardly public—information on organizational websites, promotional material, artistic expressions—and should be treated as published information and given due attribution. In other cases, the 'public' nature of the information may be more ambiguous. Some pointers that are useful to think through when making these decisions are: How does the person posting the information present themselves? Are they 'talking' to a general audience or to a specific group? Have they tried to restrict access to this information through passwords or other mechanisms? Have they tried to protect their anonymity in other ways? Forums and social networking sites, which have been one of the most frequently used sources of information in studies of patients' experiences, are often particularly sensitive.

In some cases the forum/website owners will explicitly state that researchers are not allowed to analyse the content, while in others they may warn users that any information they post is in the public domain and advise them to protect their anonymity accordingly. Even in the latter cases, it is still necessary to bear in mind that not all users will view the privacy of the information they upload in the same way and may not have read the privacy terms of the online services they are using. One potentially useful way of thinking through this is to try to balance 'group accessibility'—the public/private nature of the online space in question—and 'perceived privacy'—the level of privacy that users may think they have (King, 1996). However, even in ostensibly 'public' forums, it is necessary to carefully consider how and why the information is used: could any harm be inflicted on the user because of the research? What are the potential benefits for the user and for others? Are there any additional steps that could minimize potential problems?

Sometimes online material will be linked to particular individuals (e.g. blogs or YouTube videos) and its authors can be contacted and asked for permission to use their content. Indeed, in some cases it may be advisable to gain permission from content producers and even to post online as a researcher (e.g. to recruit people for interviews and/or find out more about the production side of sharing their experiences (Orgad, 2006)), in others this may be intrusive and disrupt the environment under study (Adams et al., 2005). When a researcher is already genuinely a member of a particular community it is necessary to balance the dual identity of being a participant and an observer, while also opening up interesting avenues for research.

Conclusion

Internet technologies provide numerous opportunities for studying and indeed enhancing how people experience and live with different health conditions. Given the current rate of technical change, the convergence of new media platforms and developments in mobile and pervasive health technologies, representations of health and illness are likely to constantly emerge in new forms and evolve online. As an increasingly e-literate population engages with online personal health records and digital health services, resulting in ever more forms of experiential data, interesting possibilities for researching experiences of health and illness will develop, raising new methodological challenges and opportunities for innovation.

In most cases Internet-based research on patient experiences has been based on 'traditional' research practices and methods that have been adapted for the online environment. More recently, 'digital methods', in which a distinction is made between the importation of 'traditional' methods and what have been termed 'natively digital' ones, have been suggested (Rogers, 2010). The use of 'digital methods' and other opportunities, such as the analysis of 'big data', including large user-generated datasets contained in social media postings, open up new vistas for researchers interested in how new media technologies interact with, shape, and are shaped by people's experiences of health and illness. At the same time, it requires the development of new skills for data capturing, management, and analysis, that are not typically provided as part of the training and methodological repertoire of people working in relation to patient experiences.

The Internet provides a vast repository of health information across a range of different conditions and in many different forms that can be analysed and used to contribute to understanding and improving patient experiences in different ways. However, it should not be treated and studied simply as a repository for experiences that can be mined by researchers, but also as an active player in contemporary healthcare in which the separation between old and new media, on- and offline, are becoming increasingly blurred. In this chapter we highlighted some of the ways you can study online representations of experiences of health and illness, and what such studies can contribute to our understanding and enhancement of these experiences. We have shown how different platforms and technologies are fascinating objects of analysis in their own right (e.g. how users of particular forums develop specific illness-related identities) as well as offer opportunities for exploring other phenomenon of relevance for how people experience healthcare services, make decisions about, and cope with different health conditions. Rather than being a static archive where patients record their experiences, the use of Internet technologies is increasingly forming part of those experiences. Indeed, for many people seeking out and sharing their experiences online is an intrinsic part of their illness experience. Yet, while, on the one hand, Internet technologies are a key player in the changing dynamics of contemporary healthcare, on the other they are being normalized, becoming part of the information infrastructure of healthcare.

Further reading

Heilferty, C.M. (2011). Ethical considerations in the study of online illness narratives: a qualitative review. *Journal of Advanced Nursing*, 67(5), 945–53.

Krippendorff, K. (2004). *Content analysis: An introduction to its methodology* (2nd edn). Thousand Oaks, CA: Sage.

Radin, P. (2006). 'To me, it's my life': medical communication, trust, and activism in cyberspace. *Social Science & Medicine*, 62(3), 591–601.

Seale, C., *et al.* (2010). Interviews and internet forums: a comparison of two sources of qualitative data. *Qualitative Health Research*, 20(5), 595–606.

Ziebland, S. and Wyke, S. (2012). Health and illness in a connected world: how might sharing experiences on the internet affect people's health? *Milbank Quarterly*, 90(2), 219–49.

References

Adair, C.E., *et al.* (2006). The internet as a source of data to support the development of a quality-of-life measure for eating disorders. *Qualitative Health Research*, 16(4), 538–46.

Adams, J., Rodham, K., and Gavin, J. (2005). Investigating the 'self' in deliberate self-harm. *Qualitative Health Research*, 15(10), 1293–309.

Armstrong, N., Koteyko, N., and Powell, J. (2012). 'Oh dear, should I really be saying that on here?': issues of identity and authority in an online diabetes community. *Health (London)*, 16(4), 347–65.

Bar-Lev, S. (2008). 'We are here to give you emotional support': performing emotions in an online HIV/AIDS support group. *Qualitative Health Research*, 18(4), 509–21.

Ess, C. (2002). *Ethical decision-making and internet research: Recommendations from the AoIR ethics working committee*. Association of Internet Researchers. [Online] Available at: <http://aoir.org/documents/ethics-guide> (accessed 8 August 2012).

Fox, N.J., Ward, K.J., and O'Rourke, A.J. (2005). Pro-anorexia, weight-loss drugs and the internet: an 'anti-recovery' explanatory model of anorexia. *Sociology of Health & Illness*, 27(7), 944–71.

Gillett, J. (2003). Media activism and internet use by people with HIV/AIDS. *Sociology of Health & Illness*, 25(6), 608–24.

Greaves, F., *et al.* (2012). Associations between web-based patient ratings and objective measures of hospital quality. *Archives of Internal Medicine*, 172, 435–6.

Harvey, K.J., *et al.* (2007). 'Am I normal?' Teenagers, sexual health and the internet. *Social Science & Medicine*, 65(4), 771–81.

Hine, C. (2005). *Virtual methods: Issues in social research on the Internet*. London: Berg Publishers.

Hobson-West, P. (2007). 'Trusting blindly can be the biggest risk of all': organised resistance to childhood vaccination in the UK. *Sociology of Health & Illness*, 29(2), 198–215.

Horne, J. and Wiggins, S. (2009). Doing being 'on the edge': managing the dilemma of being authentically suicidal in an online forum. *Sociology of Health & Illness*, 31(2), 170–84.

King, S.A. (1996). Researching internet communities: proposed ethical guidelines for the reporting of results. *The Information Society*, 12(2), 119–28.

Krippendorff, K. (2004). *Content analysis: an introduction to its methodology* (2nd edn). Thousand Oaks, CA: Sage.

O'Brien, M.R. and Clark, D. (2012). Unsolicited written narratives as a methodological genre in terminal illness. *Qualitative Health Research*, 22(2), 274–84.

Orgad, S. (2006). The cultural dimensions of online communication: a study of breast cancer patients' internet spaces. *New Media & Society*, 8(6), 877–99.

Robinson, K.M. (2001). Unsolicited narratives from the internet: a rich source of qualitative data. *Qualitative Health Research*, 11(5), 706–14.

Rogers, R. (2010). Internet research: the question of method. *Journal of Information Technology and Politics*, 7(2/3), 241–60.

Seale, C., Ziebland, S., and Charteris-Black, J. (2006). Gender, cancer experience and internet use: A comparative keyword analysis of interviews and online cancer support groups. *Social Science & Medicine*, 62(10), 2577–90,

Seale, C., *et al.* (2010). Interviews and internet forums: a comparison of two sources of qualitative data. *Qualitative Health Research*, *20*(5), 595–606.

Skea, Z.C., *et al.* (2008). 'Avoiding harm to others' considerations in relation to parental measles, mumps and rubella (MMR) vaccination discussions—an analysis of an online chat forum. *Social Science & Medicine*, *67*(9), 1382–90.

Woolgar, S. (ed.) (2002). *Virtual society? Technology, cyberbole, reality.* Oxford: Oxford University Press.

Ziebland, S. and Wyke, S. (2012). Health and illness in a connected world: how might sharing experiences on the internet affect people's health? *Milbank Quarterly*, *90*(2), 219–49.

Chapter 11

Systematic review and synthesis of qualitative research

Ruth Garside

Background

> The work which deserves, but I am afraid does not always receive, the most credit, is that in which discovery and explanation go hand in hand, in which not only are new facts presented, but their relation to old ones pointed out.
>

This chapter considers the role of systematic review and synthesis of qualitative research in evidence-based medicine (EBM), and how this may be used to illuminate what is known about patient experiences. Systematic review of quantitative research has been the cornerstone of EBM since the 1990s. EBM intends to ensure that health decisions at personal, practitioner, and policy levels are based on the best existing evidence rather than relying on tradition, experience, or opinion (which might be unreliable) or text books (likely to be out of date) (Sackett et al., 2000). Time-pressed practitioners can only keep abreast of increasing amounts of published research if presented information is thorough and unbiased. Traditional ways of reviewing literature have been charged with bias and partiality (Egger et al., 2001); articles that reflect the authors' concerns might be preferentially included, intentionally or because these are the studies of which they are aware. Central principles of systematic review, designed to minimize such bias, include methodological transparency (approaches clear and justified), and replicability (whereby another team using the same approaches would draw similar conclusions) (Centre for Reviews and Dissemination, 2008; Higgins and Green, 2008).

Initially, EBM sometimes appeared to have a restricted understanding of 'evidence', focusing on the randomized controlled trial (RCT) (Black, 1996; Morse et al., 2001; Petticrew and Roberts, 2003). Whilst non-RCT quantitative study designs were also affected, qualitative research was in particular danger of being marginalized. Indeed, qualitative research was sometimes omitted entirely from an evidence hierarchy. While understandable for reviews about the relative effects of treatments for a particular condition, it is increasingly recognized that different kinds of evidence are required to investigate different, equally pertinent questions (Petticrew and Roberts, 2003). Understanding patients' perspectives on health, illness, and services is crucial to offer appropriate support, plan acceptable services, and understand factors that might prevent or enhance effectiveness. Qualitative studies can illuminate how and why people participate in research and what patient preferences for treatment and services might be. They can help policymakers understand how and why some interventions are more successful than others, and why interventions which *can* be successful, fail to be in specific circumstances. This has helped to increase interest in methods of systematic review of qualitative research.

Novelty is prized in academic research, with researchers encouraged to establish the innovative nature of their work to secure funding or publish findings. Researchers are, however, increasingly required by editors to outline what is *already* known in the total field of interest in order to situate their work within it. It has been argued that 'formal synthesis of both quantitative and qualitative forms of research is essential to address uncertainties in many areas of healthcare' (Dixon-Woods et al., 2001). Evidence synthesis also produces original insights, requiring new analytic skills and techniques. Advocates state that they are driven:

> not by some frivolous urge to be creative about ideas or by a presumptuous desire to author a new way of thinking, but by the abiding sense that the process may yield truths that are better or more socially relevant, or more complete than those from which we currently operate (Paterson et al., 2001).

Among some qualitative researchers, systematic review and synthesis remains controversial. Its acceptance as a legitimate project might derive, at least partly, from strategic considerations: to refuse may further marginalize qualitative studies' ability to influence healthcare policy and practice (Walsh and Downe, 2005). Qualitative researchers have often failed to cite similar, relevant research, particularly outside their own discipline, leaving findings isolated, and resulting in underdeveloped concepts and theories (Campbell et al., 2003). Individual projects' findings have been described as a jigsaw puzzle which, while interesting and illuminating, offer no clue as to the relationship between the pieces and thus what the complete field might look like (Paterson et al., 2001). Synthesis of qualitative research can provide more powerful explanations through higher-order conceptualization and more broadly encompassing theories (Dixon-Woods et al., 2004). Syntheses explore findings initially appearing contradictory, that may otherwise be overlooked or ignored (Paterson et al., 2001; Greenhalgh et al., 2005). Similarities and differences in findings can be explored in terms of study participants, dates, and locations, as well as the methods used by the researchers and their disciplinary frameworks.

Through failing to optimize the use of previous findings, not synthesizing can be seen as wasteful from the perspective of the participants, who have given their time and revealed their experiences, and researchers, whose contributions add to a body of knowledge. It could be argued that there is a moral obligation to ensure that the perspectives of research participants are taken to the broadest audience and that future research builds on what is known. Synthesis also offers better value for money for funders of the original research.

The emphasis on context within qualitative research has led some to argue that findings cannot be 'generalizable' as the term is used by quantitative studies with representative samples. For others, it is merely a conflict of terminology; with results considered 'transferable' or 'applicable' when the context and approaches are described in enough detail for readers to establish whether such a context might apply to their own circumstances (Jackson and Haworth-Brockman, 2007). Generalizability can also be seen at the level of developed concepts and theories, rather than specific descriptive findings.

While systematic reviews have been the focus of EBM since inception, the inclusion of qualitative research has only gathered pace since the late 2000s. Break-through examples have demonstrated the shift in understanding about the value of qualitative research notably, in UK policymaking, the Centre for Public Health Excellence at the National Institute for Health and Clinical Excellence (NICE) which routinely includes syntheses of qualitative research to identify factors which help or hinder the success of interventions (Centre for Public Health Excellence, 2009). Limits remain: the Cochrane Collaboration, the global coordinator of systematic review evidence for healthcare interventions, only accepts qualitative syntheses which mirror questions posed by quantitative meta-analyses, rather than being valued in their own right (Higgins and Green, 2008).

Undertaking a systematic review

Debate continues about the specifics of almost all stages of systematic reviews of qualitative research. Within the policymaking arena, approaches tend to mirror those developed for quantitative research, although there is increasing recognition that differences in approach are not just possible, but desirable. Several mechanisms have been proposed for the synthesis steps of the review, some adopt a more aggregative approach (such as those developed by the Evidence for Policy and Practice Information and Co-ordinating Centre (EPPI-Centre, 2007)), others embrace more sophisticated interpretative approaches (such as meta-study and meta-ethnography (Paterson et al., 2001; Britten et al., 2002)).

Approaches to reduce bias, such and replicability and transparency, are key to the systematic review paradigm. Replicability may be a tall order and, arguably, inappropriate for an interpretive approach although it should always be clear how the theory, findings, and conclusions relate to each other. Many qualitative researchers are familiar with keeping an audit trail so that important decisions about the analysis are recorded and justified; this can also be used in syntheses.

Traditionally, systematic reviews demand pre-specified protocols to ensure transparency. These define the research question, approach to identifying, including, and appraising studies, and synthesis of their findings. These stages are outlined in the following sections: more detailed accounts can be found elsewhere (Paterson et al., 2001; Petticrew and Roberts, 2006; EPPI-Centre, 2007; Pope et al., 2007; Sandelowski and Barroso, 2007; Centre for Reviews and Dissemination, 2008; Higgins and Green, 2008). Where changes are made to the originally proposed approaches, these should be recorded and justified: this is a requirement where protocols are registered, such as the Cochrane Library.

Defining research questions

These may need to be refined iteratively through scoping searches and consultation with commissioners to ensure that the depth and breadth of the review is both meaningful and manageable. Definitions of the population and the condition or intervention of interest are specified. For reviews of RCTs, the nature of the intervention and comparator treatment is key, but this is not always useful for qualitative reviews (see Box 11.1). Areas of interest may emerge during the synthesis. A review about women's experiences of hysterectomy, for example, initially excluded research which only discussed oophorectomy, but the synthesis revealed this as an important consideration among women undergoing hysterectomy (Garside, 2008).

Box 11.1 Synthesis example 1: prevention of skin cancer

As part of NICE CPHE's development of guidance about preventing the first instance of skin cancer, a systematic review and synthesis of qualitative evidence was requested (Garside et al., 2010). Asked to identify the barriers and facilitators to adopting messages of such public health campaigns, the nature of the inclusion criteria for the review was refined iteratively as the project progressed. Our original protocol included only studies that had addressed people's experiences of particular prevention campaigns. During searching and screening, this changed to include any study of attitudes towards, and experiences of, tanning, sunburn, use of sunbeds, and protection against the sun. We found few studies that evaluated specific campaigns (n = 3) and those that did, also explored attitudes generally, making them similar to other studies that did not focus on a campaign.

The synthesis used the Health Belief Model (HBM) as an imported framework to structure the analysis (Becker, 1974). Within this, meta-ethnography techniques were drawn on to understand the findings of the included papers in relation to each other. Of the 16 included study reports, four used the HBM.

In summary, the synthesis found that adults and children generally perceived themselves at low susceptibility of developing skin cancer while its severity was seen as a minor, future risk, which would be curable if it occurred. Few participants held spurious beliefs about causes and prevention strategies. While they understood the theoretical benefits of taking preventative action, however, this was often not reflected in how they behaved. Barriers to adopting safer sun behaviour included positive perceptions of tanned skin as healthy and attractive. Covering up or applying suncream was seen as a hassle. In addition, being outdoors was itself seen as healthy, and people were less likely to protect themselves when tanning was incidental, rather than sought (such as when not at the beach).

This synthesis allowed common perceptions and misconceptions to be identified which could facilitate or act against public health messages.

Identifying literature

A search strategy for electronic databases is usually a central mechanism, for which the input of an information specialist (IS) is invaluable. Multiple databases are examined, because they index different disciplines and journals: an IS can undertake the necessary 'translation' of the search strategy. A number of filters to identify qualitative research have been developed but, as the indexing in databases is less well developed than for trials, many irrelevant hits are also returned which need to be screened (Shaw et al., 2004). Backwards and forward citation chasing of relevant papers, contact with authors in the field, and browsing are also useful ways of identifying relevant papers (Sandelowski and Barroso, 2007).

Explicit inclusion and exclusion criteria for studies

These may be refined through piloting. As well as deciding whether the synthesis aims to learn from the views of patients, health professionals, family members, and so on, considerations include whether location of research, language, date of publication, etc. will be defined. Some approaches to synthesis advocate restricting studies to those from a particular epistemological position (Jensen and Allen, 1996), while others describe specific techniques for tracing the story of research within traditions and disciplines, and also allow for these to be critiqued within the synthesis (Paterson et al., 2001; Greenhalgh et al., 2005).

Potentially includable references and abstracts are usually uploaded into reference management software (such as ENDNOTE, REFMAN) which facilitates review processes. Reviewers scan these, marking those that appear to meet inclusion criteria. It can be difficult to know from the title and abstract whether a paper should be included, so full texts of potential articles are obtained and similarly screened for inclusion. Reasons for not including any papers at this stage are recorded on a flow chart showing the number of references screened at each stage and the final numbers of included papers. It is usual for two reviewers to independently screen references and papers to avoid mistakes and discuss ambiguities.

Data extraction and quality appraisal

For each included research paper, methods, participant characteristics, and other study details are recorded in a bespoke data extraction form. Findings, in the form of key quotes, themes, concepts, and metaphors, are also recorded.

Best practice is for at least two reviewers to independently extract data so that different interpretations and understandings can be highlighted and discussed.

Each study is also usually quality appraised. While a standard stage of traditional systematic reviews, there has been considerable debate about the best approaches and, indeed, whether it is appropriate at all, given the lack of consensus between researchers working within different disciplines and traditions. Numerous checklists and guidelines have been developed; many long, and often emphasizing quite different criteria (Walsh and Downe, 2005; Sandelowski and Barroso, 2007). These require judgement and studies have shown little consensus between different reviewers using the same tool (Dixon-Woods, 2005). Despite the problems, there is agreement that some way of distinguishing high-quality studies from poor is desirable, although whether poor-quality studies should still be included in the synthesis and how, remains contested. It may be helpful to distinguish between the technical elements of reporting (whether there is enough detail reported to understand what was done in the study) and those which relate to the nature of the epistemological and ontological approach (Popay, 2008). Again, it is useful to have at least two reviewers involved in the quality appraisal to facilitate debate about the merits of particular approaches.

Analysis and synthesis

There are a number of suggested approaches to synthesizing qualitative research studies; the approach taken will relate to the review purpose and the nature of the included studies. Meta-ethnography seems to work best where papers are strongly conceptual (see Box 11.2) while a review dominated by descriptive studies may use a technique like thematic analysis. Approaches may use familiar qualitative analysis techniques (such as thematic analysis or grounded theory, see also Chapter 5) or those developed specifically for synthesis, such as meta-narrative, meta-study, or meta-ethnography (Noblit and Hare, 1988; Paterson et al., 2001; Britten et al., 2002, Campbell et al., 2003; Sandelowski and Barroso, 2003; Greenhalgh et al., 2005). Synthesis may use existing second-order concepts (the interpretations of the researchers) as the basis of the review, or may look at the detail of the individual data extracts presented in the original paper. As with any qualitative analysis, techniques to classify (or code), order, juxtapose, compare, and integrate findings are required (Popay et al., 2006). A multidisciplinary team is invaluable, particularly where papers are drawn from a number of disciplinary and theoretical frameworks.

Box 11.2 Synthesis example 2: patient experience of medicine taking

There are increasing numbers of review examples that illuminate the patient perspective. An early example tested the feasibility of using meta-ethnography, originally developed to synthesize findings of ethnographic, education studies, as a tool for synthesizing the findings of qualitative research in healthcare (Britten et al., 2002; Campbell et al., 2003) As originally outlined, it is purely an approach to synthesis, so offers no guidance about other stages of a systematic review (Noblit and Hare, 1988). These have been adapted from elsewhere. Meta-ethnography uses 'translation' to describe the analytic approach whereby findings between different studies are considered in relation to each other, and compared for similarities ('reciprocal translation'), opposing findings ('refutational translation'), and may be pieced together to form a 'line of argument' synthesis. Meta-ethnography has become a well-used approach, especially in the UK.

Pound et al. (2005) produced a meta-ethnography to describe experiences of medicine-taking in order to examine the way in which patients themselves view activities which are usually described in the clinical literature as 'compliance', 'adherence', or 'concordance' with a clinically prescribed regimen (Pound et al., 2005). The review included 37 papers which focused on patient views about taking medicine. The synthesis product was descriptive, but also resulted in a schematic model of medicine taking which captures people's reasoning behind different approaches (see Figure 11.1).

Strengths and limitations

The results of syntheses may be used by researchers, patients, health professionals, and policymakers. Qualitative synthesis can systematically identify what is known about, for example, experiences and understandings of a condition, treatment, or service or, indeed, any topic appropriate for a qualitative research approach, allowing a comprehensive understanding of a body of research. It can add weight to research on patients' experiences, can be dismissed as too anecdotal or context specific, through demonstrating that there are core issues across the field. Policymakers may be more inclined to accept findings gleaned across a number of localities, times, and groups. Increasingly, healthcare guideline development and policy uses formal syntheses.

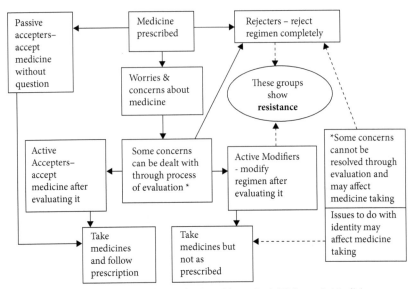

Fig. 11.1 Model of medicine taking. Reprinted from *Social Science & Medicine*, Volume 61, Issue 1, Pandora Pound et al. Resisting medicines: a synthesis of qualitative studies of medicine taking, pp. 133–55, Copyright © 2005, with permission from Elsevier, DOI: <http://dx.doi.org/10.1016/j.socscimed.2004.11.063>.

Where more conceptual methods are used, it also presents opportunities to develop more comprehensive or relevant theories.

Any systematic review is limited by the quality and scope of existing literature. Even in these cases, however, it is useful to highlight gaps, trends, or limitations in the evidence base. For example, reviews may find that little research has been done in particular groups of people or that restricted questions about a topic have dominated the literature: this may help to direct future research.

Quality appraisal remains divisive. While some qualitative researchers believe that their methods of research, and particularly analysis, should be clear and codified, others have argued that the iterative, flexible approach needed means that this may be neither feasible nor desirable (Bryman and Burgess, 1994). Some researchers view synthesis of findings from several projects as inappropriate to the epistemological underpinnings of qualitative research. It has been suggested that the uniqueness of the interaction between those informing the research and the centrality of context—historical, socio-political, intellectual—inevitably frustrates meaningful synthesis (Sandelowski et al., 1997).

Qualitative synthesis offers an opportunity for researchers to usefully inform policy, rather than remain in a rarefied academic position. The Health Development Agency has written:

> much of the methodological debate is completely unhelpful from a point of view of trying to bring about reductions in the inequalities in health, does nothing to help develop policy and practice, is a gross oversimplification of important scientific work in a range of methodological traditions, and—as a final shot—is a misrepresentation of the philosophical principles which supposedly are the origins of the so-called divide (Dixon-Woods et al., 2004).

Policymakers in the UK and beyond (see Chapter 15) are committed to understanding and prioritizing patients' experiences of healthcare; qualitative researchers who recognize the potential of synthesis both as a pragmatic technique for informing practice *and* as a theoretical tool, can perform a key role in bringing analytic understanding of the experiences of patients to a wider audience.

Further reading

Britten, N., *et al.* (2002). Using meta-ethnography to synthesise qualitative research: a worked example. *Journal of Health Services Research & Policy*, 7(4) 209–15.

Centre for Reviews and Dissemination. (2008). *Systematic reviews. CRD's guidance for undertaking reviews in health care.* York: York Publishing Services.

EPPI Centre. (2007). *EPPI-Centre methods for conducting systematic reviews.* London: EPPI-Centre, Social Science Research Unit, Institute of Education, University of London.

Petticrew, M. and Roberts, H. (2006). *Systematic reviews in the social sciences: A practical guide.* Oxford: Blackwell Publishing.

Sandelowski, M. and Barroso, J. (2007). *Handbook for synthesizing qualitative research.* New York, NY: Springer Publishing Company.

References

Becker, M. (1974). *The health belief model and personal heath behaviour.* Thorofare, NJ: Charles B. Slack.

Black, N. (1996). Why we need observational studies to evaluate the effectiveness of health care. *British Medical Journal, 312,* 1215–18.

Britten, N., *et al.* (2002). Using meta-ethnography to synthesise qualitative research: a worked example. *Journal of Health Services Research & Policy, 7,* 209–15.

Bryman, A. and Burgess, R.G. (1994). Reflections on qualitative data analysis. In: Bryman, A. and Burgess, R.G. (eds) *Analyzing qualitative data.* London: Routledge.

Campbell, R., *et al.* (2003). Evaluating meta-ethnography: a synthesis of qualitative research on lay experiences of diabetes and diabetes care. *Social Science & Medicine, 56,* 671–84.

Centre for Public Health Excellence. (2009). *Methods for the development of NICE public health guidance* (2nd edn). London: National Institute for Health and Clinical Excellence.

Centre for Reviews and Dissemination. (2008). *Systematic reviews. CRD's guidance for undertaking reviews in health care.* York: York Publishing Services.

Chalmers, I. (2001). Foreword. In: Egger, M., Smith, G.D., and Altman, D.G. (eds) *Systematic reviews in health care. Meta-analysis in context.* London: BMJ Books.

Dixon-Woods, M. (2005). *Qualitative and quantitative synthesis methods: principles and practice.* Qualitative Research & Systematic Reviews Workshop 27–29 June 2005, Oxford.

Dixon-Woods, M., *et al.* (2004). *Integrative approaches to qualitative and quantitative evidence.* London: Health Development Agency.

Dixon-Woods, M., Fitzpatrick, R., and Roberts, K. (2001). Including qualitative research in systematic reviews: opportunities and problems. *Journal of Evaluation in Clinical Practice, 7,* 125–33.

Egger, M., Smith, G.D., and Altman, D.G. (2001). *Systematic review in health care. Meta-analysis in context.* London: BMJ Books.

EPPI Centre. (2007). *EPPI-Centre methods for conducting systematic reviews.* London: EPPI-Centre, Social Science Research Unit, Institute of Education, University of London.

Garside, R. (2008). *A comparison of methods for the systematic review of qualitative research: Two examples using meta-ethnography and meta-study.* PhD thesis, University of Exeter, UK.

Garside, R., Pearson, M., and Moxham, T. (2010). What influences the uptake of information to prevent skin cancer? A systematic review and synthesis of qualitative research. *Health Education Research, 25,* 162–82.

Greenhalgh, T., *et al.* (2005). Storylines of research in diffusion of innovation: a meta-narrative approach to systematic review. *Social Science & Medicine, 61,* 417–30.

Higgins, J.P.T. and Green, S. (eds) (2008). *Cochrane handbook for systematic reviews of interventions.* Chichester: Wiley.

Jackson, B.E. and Haworth-Brockman, M.J. (2007). The quality of evidence: enhancing uptake of qualitative evidence for gender equity and health. *International Journal of Public Health, 52,* 265–6.

Jensen, L.A. and Allen, M.N. (1996). Meta-synthesis of qualitative findings. *Qualitative Health Research, 6,* 553–60.

Morse, J.M., Swanson, J.M., and Kuzel, A.J. (2001). *The nature of qualitative evidence.* Thousand Oaks, CA: Sage.

Noblit, G.W. and Hare, R.D. (1988). *Meta-ethnography: Synthesizing qualitative studies.* London: Sage.

Paterson, B., *et al.* (2001). *Meta-study of qualitative health research: A practical guide to meta-analysis and meta-synthesis.* Thousand Oaks, CA: Sage.

Petticrew, M. and Roberts, H. (2003). Evidence, hierarchies, and typologies: horses for courses. *Journal of Epidemiology and Community Health, 57,* 527–9.

Petticrew, M. and Roberts, H. (2006). *Systematic reviews in the social sciences: A practical guide.* Oxford: Blackwell Publishing.

Popay, J. (2008). *Using qualitative research to inform policy and practice*. Cardiff: ONS.

Popay, J., *et al.* (2006). *Guidance on the conduct of narrative synthesis in systematic reviews*. London: ESRC Methods Programme.

Pope, C., Mays, N., and Popay, J. (2007). *Synthesizing qualitative and quantitative health evidence*. Maidenhead: Open University Press.

Pound, P., *et al.* (2005). Resisting medicines: a synthesis of qualitative studies of medicine taking. *Social Science & Medicine, 61,* 133–55.

Sackett, D.L., *et al.* (2000). *Evidence-based medicine. How to practice and teach EBM*. Edinburgh: Churchill Livingstone.

Sandelowski, M. and Barroso, J. (2003). Toward a metasynthesis of qualitative findings on motherhood in HIV-positive women. *Research in Nursing & Health, 26,* 153–70.

Sandelowski, M. and Barroso, J. (2007). *Handbook for synthesizing qualitative research*. New York, NY: Springer Publishing Company.

Sandelowski, M., Docherty, S., and Emden, C. (1997). Qualitative metasynthesis: issues and techniques. *Research in Nursing & Health, 20,* 365–71.

Shaw, R.L. *et al.* (2004). Finding qualitative research: an evaluation of search strategies. *BMC Medical Research Methodology, 4,* 5.

Walsh, D. and Downe, S. (2005). Methodological issues in nursing research: meta-synthesis method for qualitative research: a literature review. *Journal of Advanced Nursing, 50,* 204–11.

Chapter 12

Harnessing patients' awareness of adverse reactions to the drugs they take

Claire Anderson and Andrew Herxheimer

The World Health Organization (WHO) (2008) defines adverse drug reactions (ADRs) as harmful, unintended reactions to medicines that occur at doses normally used for treatment. ADRs range in severity from mild to serious and even fatal. A side effect may appear as soon as someone starts taking a medicine. Occasionally, side effects can appear after a person has stopped taking the medicine. Some side effects are not discovered until many people have been taking the medicine for some time, often long after it has come into use. Patients need to be well informed about the nature and timing (a) of the intended effects of a medicine and (b) of its possible harmful or inconvenient effects, to enable them to weigh the expected benefits against the possible disadvantages. Knowing the effects of not taking a medicine can be as important as knowing about its benefits. Medawar and Herxheimer (2004) compared consumer reports of reactions to paroxetine with reports from professionals to the Yellow Card Scheme. They also found that reports from patients can communicate essential information which cannot be expected from professional reporters. It is important to recognize that reports from either patients or professionals lose their richness when converted to symptom codes. For example, the same authors found that some terms patients used, such as electric shock sensation associated with paroxetine, had been given less specific codes, such as paraesthesia.

On 31 December 2011 a new European directive on pharmacovigilance (European Community, 2011) signalled a very important change. It amended Directive 2001/83/EC on the community code relating to human medicines, saying that Union rules on pharmacovigilance 'should be based on the crucial role of healthcare professionals in monitoring the safety of medicines, and should take account of the fact that patients are also well placed to report suspected adverse reactions to medical products. It is therefore appropriate to facilitate the reporting of suspected adverse reactions by both … professionals and patients, and to make methods for such reporting available to them'. This directive came into force in July 2012. In May 2012, WHO published short practical guidelines on how to set up national systems for the general public to report adverse reactions to medicines (WHO, 2012).

Why pharmacovigilance matters

Pharmacovigilance is defined as the science and activities relating to the detection, assessment, understanding, and prevention of adverse effects or any other medicine-related problem (WHO, 2004). Pharmacovigilance is essential because rare, delayed, serious, and/or unexpected adverse effects often emerge only when medicines are widely used. Many countries have a pharmacovigilance system which includes spontaneous reporting, but so far few of them, for example, the Netherlands, Australia, Brazil, Canada, and Thailand, accept such reports from the general public (Avery et al., 2011). Direct reporting by consumers can help to promote their rights, and acknowledge that consumers have unique perspectives and experiences—though only if the organizations receiving the reports act on them appropriately can consumers benefit from their involvement. National drug regulators have until now failed to do so. They have seen the new European directive coming but have shown no sign that they will reorganize and improve their work.

Scurti et al. (2012) called for a more patient-centred approach to pharmacovigilance, building on the vision of Archie Cochrane outlined in 1972: 'He anticipated the present awareness of trials and epidemiology, efficacy and effectiveness, risk management and rights of patients and populations, as a continuum of complementary tools, strategies and actors to make institutions and health care systems accountable to and in dialogue with society' (Scurti et al., 2012, p. 12). They note 'groups of patients and their families are perfectly able and motivated to produce pertinent information on how treatments (beyond this or that molecule) affect the autonomy of their lives with greater reliability and more direct implications for timely adjustments of prescribing behaviours'.

In most countries the national drug regulatory agency is responsible for monitoring the (un)safety of medicines; in the UK this is the Medicines and Healthcare products Regulatory Agency (MHRA). It collects reports of suspected ADRs from health professionals and consumers. The information from Yellow Cards is entered into a database (MHRA, 2012). The reports are evaluated each week to look for previously unidentified hazards and other new information on the side effects of medicines. Since 2005, patients in the UK have used Yellow Card reporting online, by telephone, or on paper; forms are available from general practitioner (GP) surgeries, pharmacies, and the Internet.

Other sources of patients' reports of adverse events

Patients' reports of adverse events related to illness or treatment were few until the advent of the Internet. A notable pioneering bibliography was Aronson's *Patients' Tales,* begun in 1999, and now an active and expanding website (<http://www.patientstales.org>). It lists books written about illnesses by the people who experienced them. Most of them are single-volume autobiographical accounts, but the list also includes some books of essays and single essays published in books. Some entries include a commentary on the book.

In the last 15 years the Internet has spawned many new ways of collecting and publishing personal experiences of medicines. The aims and motives range from the wish to share experiences with others and finding help and support, to doing systematic research on them, and assembling reliable information for everybody. Some chat rooms and discussion groups, particularly those of patient groups, focus on particular diseases, others on particular drugs or drug groups. Many are part of or linked with a site offering users information and education on a condition or disease, and use personal experiences as illustrations. An unplanned early collection followed the BBC television programme 'Secrets of Seroxat': its makers received almost 1,400 emails responding to it, many people reporting their own experiences. They were not published but could be analysed and compared with other reports (Medawar et al., 2002)

Some are *publicly funded*, like <http://www.tellingstories.nhs.uk>, a site of the National Genetics Education and Development Centre. The Dutch site <http://www.meldpuntmedicijnen.nl>, funded by the Ministry of Health, invites brief reports from users. Many are *charities*, for example, DIPEx, whose primary work is to collect narratives showing as nearly as possible the full range of experiences of all kinds of illnesses and health problems (not just of treatments). The Health Experiences Research Group at the University of Oxford does the qualitative research for its collections on <http://Healthtalkonline. org> and <http://Youthhealthtalk.org>; the charity runs the websites.

A new international site on the harms of prescription medicines, <http://www.RxISK.org>, is still being built. It is compendious, ambitious, and critical. Some sites are explicitly *for profit*, for example, <http://www.PatientsLikeMe. com> in the US 'is a for-profit company (with a not-just-for-profit attitude). Every partnership we develop must bring us closer to aligning patient and industry interests. Our end goal is improved patient care and quality of life'. A newer Dutch example is <http://www.mijnmedicijn.nl> [my medicine], with similar sites called <http://www.meamedica.de> in Germany, France, Belgium, Switzerland, and Austria; others in Spain and Italy will follow.

Documentary analysis of patient reports of adverse drug reactions

Avery's group used documentary analysis to examine patients' Yellow Card reports and assess the richness of their data in comparison with those from professionals (Avery et al., 2011). They analysed reports from patients and professionals, selecting a wide range of different types of report. Focusing on the free text describing the ADRs, they analysed the content of 230 patients' and 179 professionals' reports in detail. A range of different categories and reactions from Yellow Card reports were sampled.

In a pilot sample of ten reports from patients and ten from professionals' reports, categories were identified from the descriptions in the free-text field. The categories were identified inductively through iterative reading of the texts and discussion among researchers. Once the main data analysis began, some categories were refined to improve their precision or widen their definition. For example, for text about clinical 'signs' it was decided to focus on 'physical signs observed by professionals' since otherwise symptoms and signs could not be clearly separated. Where texts noted that an ADR had improved on stopping a drug, they turned out to include examples of improvement when a dose had been reduced, so the definition was widened to include this possibility. The categories were stable early in the analysis, allowing quantification across the sample. In broad terms, the categories covered:

- description of the problem
- impact of the adverse reaction on the patient
- descriptions of the possible association between the drug and adverse effects
- the patient's background medical history
- what the patient did
- involvement of professionals.

In addition, fields were created to allow assessment of other features of the reports, such as ambiguities or possible recording errors. The elaborateness of the accounts was judged qualitatively, scoring them as: 0, no narrative; 1, scant narrative; 2, moderately elaborate; 3, very elaborate. It was also noted whether the symptoms were presented as extreme. A researcher read each ADR report and noted the presence of information in the various categories. Data were entered into Microsoft Excel and double checked. The number and percentage of reports containing each information item was calculated for the patients' and the professionals' reports.

A detailed qualitative content analysis was then done by iteratively reading the data in each category, with particular reference to the categories where the frequency in reports from patients and professionals differed substantially. The data were read by one researcher, entered into the NVivo software and coded. Two other researchers checked and verified the initial categories identified. Disagreement over the codes or the interpretation of the reports were discussed and reviewed. The analysis used the technique of constant comparison and the identification of outlying cases (Pope et al., 2000). The transcripts were read repeatedly and discussed in relation to the key categories identified. As well as looking for differences between patients' and professionals' reports, those issues that the content analysis had highlighted were categorized. Particular types of reactions that seemed to be reported at different rates by patients and professionals were also categorized, for example, electric shock sensations and suicidal ideation.

Both patients (93%) and professionals (78%) described symptoms of ADRs, but patients' reports were much more detailed and extensive. Patients noted much more often than professionals how extreme and how frightening signs and symptoms were.

Reports about electric shock syndrome and antidepressants illustrate how if such a new serious and unpleasant adverse effect were to occur from a drug in the future, patients' reports could contribute to pharmacovigilance and to understanding of an ADR. Forty-seven per cent of patients' reports and 14% of professionals' reports about the antidepressants citalopram, paroxetine, and venlafaxine included descriptions of 'electric shock feelings' or similar reactions. Patients' reports of this particular symptom tend to stress its severity. They were much more vivid, comparing this reaction to other extreme experiences and stressing its intensity. Several professionals listed electric shocks as a reaction, but only one in the sample described it in more detail, quoting the patient's own description.

The in-depth qualitative analysis of the reports proved to be a very useful method and showed the richness of accounts of ADRs from patients, with many detailed and elaborate descriptions of suspected reactions. Patients described suspected ADRs in detail, attributing reactions to specific medicines, and gave information useful for assessing causality. Patient reports also noted why drugs had been prescribed, reasons for reporting, how patients identified the ADR, and what professionals had said. Particularly striking were patients' reports, often about central nervous system drugs, which were extremely distressing, and sometimes frightening. Reports also vividly described the effects of suspected ADRs on patients' lives, including serious disruption of social and occupational functioning and emotional effects. By contrast, professionals' comments on the effects of ADRs on patients' lives were usually brief and rarely illustrated the profound impact on normal functioning noted by patients.

Applications of the approach

Gross under-reporting by professionals and under-recognition of adverse effects is a major reason why consumer reporting has been accepted. Harms are often unrecognized, ignored, denied, hidden, or attributed to other causes. It has often been hard to persuade regulators and even more so the pharmaceutical industry that a particular harm has occurred. To convince them, all available research methods to demonstrate these effects must be fully used and combined.

Thorough analyses require detailed descriptions, but regulators and companies appear to have made little effort to get them. Reports are rarely followed up. However, regulators and companies resist disclosing even the details they have—often citing data protection and/or commercial confidentiality. The protection of public health and patients should always come first.

Many have acknowledged that patient ADR reporting is the *right* thing to do and will enhance pharmacovigilance (WHO, 2000; van Grootheest and de Jong-van den Berg, 2004; George, 2006), though the specific value of ADR reports from patients has not been clear. Proponents have highlighted potential benefits from patient reporting of ADRs (Jarernsiripornkul et al., 2003; Foster et al., 2007; de Langen et al., 2008), but others doubted that consumers can distinguish suspect ADRs from problems associated with the condition being treated (van Grootheest et al., 2003); feared that new drug safety issues would be swamped by reports of minor and well-known ADRs; that it would cost too much; that campaigning groups might influence signal generation (Metters, 2004); and perceived undermining of professionals' status (Waller, 2006).

A major reason for advocating consumer reporting (Anonymous, 2001) was that many ADRs that patients reported to GPs were not passed to the MHRA, or even noted in medical records (Jarernsiripornkul et al., 1998, 2002). Little is known about why patients report adverse reactions to schemes like the UK's Yellow Card Scheme, but a Dutch study found that patients report an ADR when they feel their doctor has not acknowledged their concerns (van Grootheest and de Jong-van den Berg, 2004). Van Hunsel et al. (2010a, 2010b,) explored why patients reported ADRs. They did so mainly because of their severity and the wish to share their experiences.

A Health Action International review noted that ADR reports from patients give much more detail and clearer descriptions than those from professionals (Herxheimer et al., 2010)—those who choose to report want to explain their experiences. A UK study (Avery et al., 2011) on patient reporting of ADRs to the Yellow Card Scheme confirmed this, finding that their reports contained more suspected ADRs per report than those from professionals, and described reactions in more detail. The proportion of reports categorized as 'serious' was similar, the patterns of drugs and reactions reported differed. Patient reports were richer in their descriptions of reactions than those from professionals, and more often noted the effects of ADRs on patients' lives. Combining patients' and professionals' reports generated more potential signals than professionals' reports alone. Most patient reporters found reporting fairly easy, but they suggested improvements to the scheme, including greater publicity and the redesign of Internet and paper-based reporting systems. The study concluded that patient reporting of suspected ADRs can add value to pharmacovigilance by: reporting different types of drugs and reactions than those professionals report; generating new potential signals; and describing suspected ADRs in enough detail to give useful information on likely causality and impact on patients' lives. The findings justified further promotion of patient reporting to the Yellow Card Scheme, and improving current reporting systems.

Strengths and limitations of harnessing patients' reports of adverse drug reactions (ADRs)

Avery et al. (2011) focused on the medicines most commonly reported by patients and those the MHRA had classified as 'black triangle' drugs. For these groups of drugs the data were relatively ample. For reports of medicines bought over the counter and complementary medicines reports from professionals are few; even from patients the numbers were small. Other methods, perhaps including interviews and surveys, might be needed to supplement documentary analysis.

In the study we used as an example (Avery et al., 2011) for some categories, such as text indicating the impact of the suspected ADR on the patient, the stark contrast between patients' and professionals' reports clearly represents genuine differences. For other categories, such as text indicating temporal relationships between medicines and suspected ADRs, differences were less and did not consider information available in other fields on the Yellow Card database. The data were carefully checked, the reports reread several times, and discordant cases sought out to counter possible biases.

Conclusion

Patients can give useful information for detailed pharmacovigilance assessment and for illuminating the emotional, social, and occupational impact of suspected ADRs. This could not only help to identify new ADRs, but also to help assess intensively monitored drugs in more detail or investigate drug–ADR pairings of interest.

Direct reporting by patients has highlighted the burden of ADRs on patients' lives and yet there are differences between what patients and regulatory authorities consider serious. The concurrence, or disparity, of views between patients and regulatory authorities needs exploration because current regulatory assessment of seriousness seems likely to miss important reactions that can very seriously affect people's lives. An example is electric shock sensations associated with SSRI withdrawal, which came to light through analysis of patient reports to the media (Medawar and Herxheimer, 2003).

Especially for intensively monitored drugs, close reading of reports therefore remains an essential task for regulators. An earlier review of patient reporting of ADRs (Blenkinsopp et al., 2007) concluded that poor quality of reports had not been a problem in any of the countries with a patient reporting system. Van Grootheest's group (2004) state that the quality of the *report* should be distinguished from that of the *clinical judgement* about the meaning of the ADR: to make a report useful it needs a description of the adverse reaction, its time of onset, the drug involved and concomitant medication, duration of drug use, including dates of starting and stopping, and any other relevant information. Most of their patient reports included this information.

Quality of the judgement relates to whether patients can distinguish drug-related complaints from other problems, for example, disease-related complaints (van Grootheest and de Jong-van den Berg, 2004). Many patients in the Avery et al. study seemed able to differentiate between symptoms of disease and ADRs, and some explained how they did it.

Spontaneous direct reporting has important benefits beyond pharmacovigilance: it allows greater patient participation and supports it. This fits doctors' expectations that patients agree to drug regimens and take the medicines. In the process, patients learn how to manage their medicines and to communicate more effectively with doctors, pharmacists, and nurses.

Reporting is both an expression of and a contribution to 'health literacy'. It is a learning experience which encourages reflection and self-expression, and should become an important informal part of education, especially on health matters. Patients' and consumers' reports describe the burden of ADRs for individuals, a major component of health that is missing from public health estimates of disease burden and iatrogenic effects in populations. This is a key gain in understanding. National pharmacovigilance systems must adapt their ways of working to enable them to deal appropriately with reports from consumers. Relevant staff will need training in interpreting and coding the more narrative reports from consumers, and learn how to respond to them when necessary.

Patients are becoming used to sharing and comparing their experiences, including those about ADRs. Although documentary analysis of the actual reports proved to be a very useful method, the Internet is also a valuable source and has enabled researchers to harness the power of crowd sourcing to examine adverse effects.

Further reading

Avery A.J., *et al.* (2011). Evaluation of patient reporting of adverse drug reactions to the UK 'Yellow Card Scheme': literature review, descriptive and qualitative analyses, and questionnaire surveys. *Health Technology Assessment, 15*(20), 1–234.

Herxheimer A., Crombag M., and Alves T. (2010). *Adverse drug reactions: A twelve-country survey & literature review. HAI briefing paper.* Available at: <http://www.haiweb.org/14012010/14Jan2010ReportDirectPatientReportingofADRsFINAL.pdf> (accessed 21 August 2012).

Medawar C. and Herxheimer A. (2003/2004). A comparison of adverse drug reaction reports from professionals and users, relating to risk of dependence and suicidal behaviour with paroxetine. *International Journal of Risk and Safety in Medicine, 15*, 5–19.

WHO. (2012). *Safety monitoring of medicinal products: Reporting system for the general public.* Geneva: WHO. Available at: <http://apps.who.int/medicinedocs/en/m/abstract/Js19132en/> (accessed 21 August 2012).

References

Anonymous (2001). UK call for patient adverse drug reaction reporting. *Script, 2634*, 4.

Avery, A.J., *et al.* (2011). Evaluation of patient reporting of adverse drug reactions to the UK 'Yellow Card Scheme': literature review, descriptive and qualitative analyses, and questionnaire surveys. *Health Technology Assessment, 15*(20), 1–234.

Blenkinsopp, A., *et al.* (2007). Patient reporting of suspected adverse drug reactions: a review of published literature and international experience. *British Journal of Clinical Pharmacology, 63*, 148–57.

de Langen, J., *et al.* (2008). Adverse drug reaction reporting by patients in the Netherlands: three years of experience. *Drug Safety, 31*, 515–24.

European Community. (2011). Directive 2010/84/EU of the European Parliament and of the Council. *Official Journal of the European Union, 31 December.* Available at: <http://ec.europa.eu/health/files/eudralex/vol-1/dir_2010_84/dir_2010_84_en.pdf> (accessed 21 August 2012).

Foster, J.M., van der Molen, T., and de Jong-van den Berg, L. (2007). Patient reporting of side effects may provide an important source of information in clinical practice. *European Journal of Clinical Pharmacology, 63*, 979–80.

George, C. (2006). *Reporting adverse drug reactions. A guide for healthcare professionals.* London: British Medical Association. Available at <http://www.isoponline.org/documents/news/BMAreport.pdf> (accessed 21 August 2012)

Herxheimer, A., Crombag, M. and Alves, T. (2010). *Adverse drug reactions: A twelve-country survey & literature review. HAI briefing paper.* Available at <http://www.haiweb.org/14012010/14Jan2010ReportDirectPatientReportingofADRsFINAL.pdf> (accessed 21 August 2012)

Jarernsiripornkul, N., *et al.* (2002). Patient reporting of potential adverse drug reactions: a methodological study. *British Journal of Clinical Pharmacology, 53,* 318–25.

Jarernsiripornkul, N., *et al.* (2003). Patient reporting of adverse drug reactions: useful information for pain management? *European Journal of Pain, 7,* 219–24.

Jarernsiripornkul, N., *et al.* (1998). Pharmacist-assisted patient reporting of adverse drug reactions. *Pharmaceutical Journal, 261,* R33.

Medawar, C. and Herxheimer, A. (2003/2004). A comparison of adverse drug reaction reports from professionals and users, relating to risk of dependence and suicidal behaviour with paroxetine. *International Journal of Risk and Safety in Medicine, 15,* 5–19.

Medawar, C., *et al.* (2002). Paroxetine, *PANORAMA* and user reporting of ADRs: consumer intelligence matters in clinical practice and post-marketing drug surveillance. *International Journal of Risk and Safety in Medicine, 15*(4), 161–9.

Metters, J. (2004). *Report of an independent review of access to the Yellow Card Scheme.* London: The Stationery Office. Available at: <http://www.mhra.gov.uk/home/groups/comms-ic/.../con2015008.pdf> (accessed 21 August 2012).

MHRA. (2012). *Yellow Card Scheme: Frequently asked questions on patient reporting.* [Online] Available at: <http://www.mhra.gov.uk/Safetyinformation/Reportingsafetyproblems/Reportingsuspectedadversedrugreactions/Patientreporting/Patientinformation/index.htm> (accessed 21 August 2012).

Pope, C., Ziebland, S., and Mays, N. (2000). Qualitative research in health care: analysing qualitative data. *British Medical Journal, 320,* 114–16.

Scurti, V., Romero, M., and Tognoni, G. (2012). A plea for a more epidemiological and patient-oriented pharmacovigilance. *European Journal of Clinical Pharmacology, 68,* 11–19.

van Grootheest, K. and de Jong-van den Berg, L. (2004). Review: patients' role in reporting adverse drug reactions. *Expert Opinion on Drug Safety. 3,* 363–8.

van Grootheest, K., de Graaf, L., and de Jong-van den Berg, L. (2003). Consumer adverse drug reaction reporting: a new step in pharmacovigilance? *Drug Safety, 26,* 211–17.

van Hunsel, F., *et al.* (2010a) Motives for reporting adverse drug reactions by patient-reporters in the Netherlands. *European Journal of Clinical Pharmacology, 66,* 1143–50.

van Hunsel, F.P., *et al.* (2010b). What motivates patients to report an adverse drug reaction? *Annals of Pharmacotherapy, 44,* 936–7.

Waller, P.C. (2006). Making the most of spontaneous adverse drug reaction reporting. *Basic & Clinical Pharmacology & Toxicology, 98,* 320–3.

WHO. (2000). Consumer reporting of adverse drug reactions. *WHO Drug Information, 14,* 211–15. Available at: <http://apps.who.int/medicinedocs/en/d/Js2201e/1.html>.

WHO. (2004). *Pharmacovigilance: Ensuring the safe use of medicines.* Geneva: WHO. Available at: <http://apps.who.int/medicinedocs/pdf/s6164e/s6164e.pdf> (accessed 21 August 2012).

WHO. (2008). *Medicines: Safety of medicines—adverse drug reactions. Fact sheet N°293.* [Online] <http://www.who.int/mediacentre/factsheets/fs293/en/> (accessed 21 August 2012).

WHO. (2012). *Safety monitoring of medicinal products: Reporting system for the general public.* Geneva: WHO. Available at <http://apps.who.int/medicinedocs/en/m/abstract/Js19132en/> (accessed 21 August 2012).

Chapter 13

Engagement and inclusivity in researching patients' experiences

Sara Ryan

Whilst there is increasing recognition of the importance of studying patients' experiences in health research, the inclusion of some 'seldom heard', or 'socially excluded' groups, remains an ongoing challenge. We often struggle to know how to be fully inclusive given the tensions and constraints created by the assumptions and practices of researchers, funders, ethics committees, health and policymakers, and academia. Some groups, such as people with learning difficulties, sex workers, illicit drug users, prison, homeless, or traveller populations, are often left out of health research, unless the focus of the study is the experiences of that particular group. These omissions leave our understanding of patients' experiences incomplete (see Figure 13.1).

In this chapter I begin with a critical assessment of what constitutes a 'seldom heard', or 'socially excluded' group. I then explore the key dimensions to

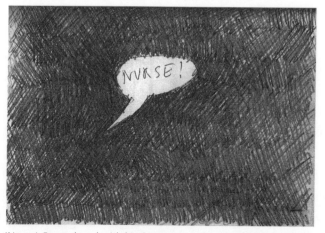

Fig. 13.1 'Nurse'. Reproduced with kind permission from Nick Wadley, *Man + Doctor*, Dalkey Archive Press, London, UK, Copyright© 2012 Nick Wadley.

facilitating inclusive research. These are summarized as: assumptions, access, time and resources, and flexible research methods. Methodological and substantive questions are raised about the expected shape and form that 'patient experience' research can take, and how this may fit into accepted standards of robust research.

What are seldom heard groups?

The need to engage with 'seldom heard' or 'socially excluded' groups has long been recognized in health and social science research. There has been a shift away from the use of the term 'hard to reach' because it suggests that the problem with engagement lies with the group, rather than the researchers (Begum, 2005). Recent UK government policy focuses on 'socially excluded' groups in health services and research (see, for example, Inclusion Health (Cabinet Office, 2010)) comprising the long-term unemployed, people experiencing domestic violence, care leavers, and ethnic minority groups. More commonly, the focus is on those considered to be most vulnerable such as homeless people, traveller groups, sex workers, and people with learning disabilities (Department of Health, 2010).

Of course these groups overlap: different dimensions of identity, including socio-economic class, ethnicity, age, and sexuality, intersect and inform people's experiences (McCall, 2005). Some of these dimensions may be more salient to the individual, while others may have more salience for their family, friends, or broader groups. For example, in a recent study exploring the experiences of people diagnosed with autism, I was contacted by family members or support workers who passed the study information to people they thought would be interested. Some of these potential participants contacted me to say that, as they were not on the autism spectrum, the study was not relevant to them. A further example is provided by Garland et al. (2006), who argue that the use of broad ethnic categories can subsume distinct communities under the broader categorization of, for example 'Black' or 'Asian'. It is important to recognize differences both between and within groups when considering how certain groups are excluded from health research. In the following section, 'Enabling inclusion', I explore some of the key dimensions of inclusive research and discuss strategies to enable inclusion.

Enabling inclusion

Assumptions

Some people are explicitly excluded at the start of a study by researchers, funders, or ethics committees because of assumptions about the 'type' of people they are. Exclusion from research often reflects a lack of awareness, understanding, and, in some cases, prejudice in mainstream society. For example:

- People with learning difficulties are often discounted from recruitment because of assumptions about their ability to understand the research process and give informed consent (Nind, 2009).

- Researchers may suspect that people who are very young, very elderly, or classified as having learning difficulties may be troublesome to include, and may doubt whether their contribution to the research will be worthwhile.

- Ethics committees may request additional layers of approval for people perceived as vulnerable due to their age or diagnosis. In some respects, this effectively grants permission to researchers to not engage with particular people.

Overcoming these often deeply embedded assumptions is challenging. Within disability studies, there has been a strong movement towards participatory and emancipatory approaches that seek to involve disabled people within the research process (see, for example, Walmsley (2001, 2004)). This has a political dimension and is intertwined with the self-advocacy movement (see, for example, Goodley (2000)). While these solutions do not necessarily challenge the assumptions of the research community, they can facilitate a deeper understanding of the experiences of disabled people. The use of peer interviewers has also been an effective strategy in other areas. For example, Benoit et al. (2005) used what they term 'a community academic collaborative approach' in their research on the sex industry. They recruited and trained ten research assistants who, as former sex workers, were able to draw on their insider knowledge of the sex trade during recruitment and data collection. These authors conclude that the research would not have been possible without this collaborative design.

Even when 'service users' are not engaged as part of the fieldwork research team it is increasingly common practice to include a patient representative as a co-applicant on grant applications. Patients also now routinely contribute to project steering groups. In this capacity they may advise on appropriate wording of recruitment materials and suggest innovative routes to recruit people from seldom heard groups. A shift towards user involvement is apparent internationally, with a growing commitment in many countries to transform research practice through service user involvement in setting the research agenda, as well as participating as advisers and co-researchers (Morrow et al., 2012).

Access

Some socially excluded groups may have complex needs or chaotic lives that make it challenging to find them (Dickson-Swift, 2005). Others may not want to be found by researchers. They may distrust or avoid researchers, sometimes because of the nature of their activities (for example, sex workers, gang members, or illicit drug users). Misunderstandings between researchers and the research population can be created by the cultural distance between researchers and potential participants (Rugkasa and Canvin, 2011). More generally, people may simply not want to take part.

In qualitative studies which seek a diverse sample, a flexible strategy can help to facilitate access. Snowball sampling, which involves asking people who have taken part in the study if they know of anyone else who may want to participate, can be an effective approach (Atkinson and Flint, 2001). Initial contacts can be achieved in a range of ways including newspaper advertisements, social media, employing an insider, community links, service contacts, or hanging out in places used by the particular group. McCormack et al. (2012) literally took to the streets, shouting for participants after the recruitment strategy in their study exploring the experiences of bisexual men, failed. They found this spontaneous innovation successful in producing a diverse sample, and also encouraged engagement from people who were unsure whether they fitted the study criteria.

Gatekeepers, including community workers, general practitioners, local voluntary groups, support workers, and carers, can help the researcher to access participants, although gaining the cooperation of the gatekeepers may take some time. Steel (2005, p. 26) recommends 'a tenacious, proactive yet sensitive approach' that involves a readiness to explain the purpose of the research, openly and honestly.

Time and resources

Meaningful inclusion can take extra time and needs to be considered at each stage of the research process. Preparation and groundwork is needed in designing the study and thinking about appropriate methods. It may be valuable to spend time within the research field and become familiar with the area. For example, in research I conducted on health experiences of people with a Jewish background, I spent time with families in a North London community in the UK, and participated in Jewish observances such as Shabbat and Purim. This enabled me to develop some familiarity with, and understanding of, Jewish culture, as well as to meet potential participants and develop trust and rapport.

Preparation and groundwork is also necessary to construct a thorough and convincing argument to include participants who may be perceived as vulnerable. Ethics committees are properly concerned to protect patients and the public, and it is important to demonstrate an awareness of and understanding of the potential challenges inclusive research can involve. A failure to do this can lead to either a lengthy process of re-submission, or a decision that the efforts required to be inclusive are not worth making. Finding effective ways of reporting the research findings is important (see, for example, Keen and Todres (2007))) ethically and strategically; since relationships in the community will be much better for researchers who avoid acting in a 'parasitic' manner by collecting data and then disappearing (Booth and Booth, 1994).

The structure of research projects can create challenges for participation. Public and voluntary sector funders and ethics committees require timetables and clear research protocols. Studies which do not allocate sufficient resources to designing research tools and recruitment procedures, and fostering relationships with contacts and gatekeepers, are unlikely to achieve wide and representative engagement. Involving, or appointing, researchers who have an established track record in research with particular seldom heard groups is likely to help.

Communication can seem difficult when trying to include people with language or cognitive problems (Lloyd et al., 2006; Tuffrey-Wijne et al., 2008). At the same time, the way in which researchers communicate, both verbally and through the use of written materials such as information sheets, can be problematic (Howard et al., 2009). Adapting standardized information sheets, using large font or pictures, personalized information, and the use of different formats (audio or video recorded versions) can ease some of these challenges (Cameron and Murphy, 2007; Oliver-Africano et al., 2010). Training may be needed to help researchers assess whether people have the mental capacity to fully understand what is involved in taking part in the research. According to the UK Mental Capacity Act 2005, capacity should be assumed, unless it is proved otherwise. This shift in emphasis should lead to the inclusion of more people in research although the safeguarding of participants remains a central consideration.

The use of relevant languages is important both in the provision of information about the study and throughout the research process. Good practice in translating questionnaires and research materials includes 'back-translation' (Rugkasa and Canvin, 2011). Using interpreters, learning a new language, and 'back' translating materials can be expensive and time-consuming. Greenhalgh (Chapter 7) used bilingual facilitators to run storytelling groups, but the researcher/observers had to rely on translations. She suggests that this allowed participants to exercise some control over what was translated and thus what contributed to the research. Stevenson (Chapter 4) notes that misunderstandings are also common when English is spoken (but not as a first language) and the participant prefers not to use an interpreter. Literacy levels vary across different populations; slight shifts in practice, such as allowing audio rather than written consent, can ease inclusion.

The need to minimize the burden on participants is particularly important for people with complex health needs or chaotic lives. Researchers should remain thoughtful, sensitive, and reflexive throughout the research study. Accessible meeting places, shorter visits to reduce fatigue or burden, willingness to reschedule or postpone appointments, and help with transport or childcare costs can all enable inclusion (Meadows et al., 2003).

Payment, or some form of compensation, has been used to widen participation but remains the subject of discussion and debate. Some argue that payment is necessary to facilitate inclusion. Others express concern that incentives can involve coercion, alter the altruistic foundations of the research paradigm or conflict with the receipt of benefits or allowances (Rugkasa and Canvin, 2011). Martinez-Ebers (1997) studied the effects of incentives on the response rates and composition of Latino groups in panel surveys in the USA. She found payment vital to increase participation rates without affecting responses to subjective questions. Of course, the type and purpose of the research is important here. In focus group studies, for example (see Chapter 6), compensation is routinely offered.

Methods

Choice of methods is an obvious consideration in inclusive research and, again, flexibility is key to effective engagement. Questionnaires or interview schedules may need to be adapted or may not be appropriate. For example, some learning disabled people may not understand complex questions or abstract concepts (Lloyd et al., 2006). Others may not be able to articulate their experiences in conventional ways in interviews. Our expectations of what health experience data 'look like' may need to be redefined. For example, concerns have been raised about incoherent speech and meaningless responses (Lloyd et al., 2006) but these concerns may relate to our perceptions of what data look like, rather than the participant's ability to convey their experiences (Aldridge, 2007).

Hyden and Brockmeier (2008) introduces the idea of broken and vicarious voices in a discussion around what researchers can do when a person lacks a voice. He identifies three possible relationships, supportive, supplementary, and substitution, between the 'authorial' voice, of the person whose narrative it is, and the 'vicarious' voice, the third person helping them tell their story. Supportive narration may include asking relevant questions, jogging memory, and encouraging the narrator. Supplementary narration involves the third person adding to the story and filling gaps with their own knowledge. This relationship involves some tension over whose authorial voice is being heard. Substitution is when others tell stories about the person who is unable to talk or articulate their experiences using other methods. Hyden illustrates this relationship with the example of Nelson (2001) whose family narrates on behalf of her sister, Carla who was born with hydrocephaly and died before she was two years old. Much of Kittay's work about her daughter Sesha, who has cerebral palsy, is also a form of substitution narrative (e.g. Kittay, 1999). Both Kittay and Nelson's writing provide Carla and Sesha with an identity and acknowledge both girls as people worthy of respect. Hyden concludes that we should maybe consider narration as an endeavour involving different voices, rather than individual storytellers.

Adaptations to methods may only emerge as necessary during the research process. In my autism research, it became apparent early on that participants found abstract questions uncomfortable and the intended, narrative interview, approach (Chapter 5) might be inappropriate. A more structured question and answer format was used for subsequent interviews. In another example, a woman contacted me to hear more about the research. After reading the information sheet, she emailed that she couldn't take part because she struggled to find the words to say during face-to-face interaction. The study design specified in-depth, face-to-face interviews but we were keen to include her perspective. I suggested doing the interview by email and she was delighted. Her hesitant, early contact, developed into a rich, detailed, and insightful account of her experiences via email exchange, see verbatim extract (Box 13.1).

Other examples of innovations to widen participation include Morse's (2002) PhD student who asked a farmer whose son had died to record his experiences

Box 13.1 Email interview exchange

I am doing an OU degree at the moment—science—and it is amazing and is keeping me safe at the moment—a constant that keeps me grounded when everything else is changing and frightening. My allotment is good— peaceful and beautiful with frogs, toads, fox,—I have a grassy area which I mow and beds of veg that I share with the wildlife (only as much as I say—I plant more than I need so we can share but if they get greedy then I cover the food!) as it is there home I am cultivating for me—I have big trees that were there before I got there and it screens me from the other allotments so it could be anywhere. The children from school come and visit in the summer to see the pond and guess the veg and even the most disruptive child is calm and understands that they are a guest of the wildlife and so am I.

on a tape recorder while he was walking around the farm. Sadness overcame him when asked to talk about it in an interview. Lu et al. (2005) in their study of people with AIDS in rural China also invited a participant to record his story in his own time. Walking interviews have been used in ethnography and can help participants to articulate their experiences more comfortably (Emmell and Clark, 2009), as can offering participants the opportunity to be interviewed with a friend or partner, rather than individually (Morris, 2001).

Photographic methods, visual methods, storytelling, drama, poetry, digital storytelling, and the use of social media and Web 2.0 have all been used to broaden research participation (Liamputtong, 2007). Talking Mats, which involve the use of symbols and pictures on a Velcro mat, can enable people with severe learning disabilities to take part in research (Murphy and Cameron, 2005). Questions remain about how to integrate and analyse some of these more experimental approaches remain and relate to more philosophical epistemological debates around the use of research methods.

Limitations to inclusion

In this chapter, I have discussed ways to increase meaningful inclusion in researching patients' experiences. However, it is important for the research community to recognize that some people may have their own good reasons for not wanting to engage with research. This can be compensated for, to some extent, in surveys by using oversampling weighting techniques (Chapter 9). There has been relatively little consideration of the costs associated with inclusive research (Beadle-Brown et al., 2012) and how we balance costly approaches and potential returns in terms of richness and diversity of data (Thompson and Phillips, 2007). Some of the suggestions detailed in this chapter are, effectively, quick wins. For example, adapting some methods, such as using email rather than a face-to-face setting, is unlikely to involve additional costs and may even be cheaper than collecting and transcribing interviews. Other suggestions, such as the creation of new methods, or increasing the time spent on fieldwork, may be more costly. It is important for researchers to remain reflexive, report limitations in the diversity of their samples, and consider what effect exclusion might have on the reach of their findings.

Conclusions

Much of the problem of including lies with assumptions about the perceived ability or competence of people to contribute to research. We have particular ideas and expectations about the shape and form of health experience research. This has led to a type of apartheid in research where people from seldom heard groups are engaged in research studies focusing only on the seldom heard groups. (So we ignore the health experiences of people with learning disabilities or sex workers or intravenous drug users.)

The keys to inclusive research are time, resources, and sensitivity. Realistic costings and timescales must be part of research proposals and should be reported more (Beadle-Brown et al., 2012). Within our own Health Experiences Research Group, in 2012 an average of £6,000 is included in research proposals to cover costs of recruitment, interpreters, and translation in qualitative interview studies of approximately 40 participants aiming for maximum variation in a UK population. Researchers may need training to assess capacity to consent and to approach vulnerable groups sensitively and appropriately. Ethics committees and funders might encourage consideration of how to include vulnerable groups rather than accepting the idea that they should be excluded from research (McCormack et al., 2012). The use of non-traditional methods of data collection, including visual methods, dramas, storytelling, and walking interviews, are increasingly being used to widen research participation (Liamputtong, 2007). This should be welcomed by public and voluntary sector funders and by ethics committees. The political imperative of reaching excluded groups and enabling their participation in shaping and reporting the outcomes of health and social care will not be achieved if patient experiences research fails to engage with and include all sectors of society and service users.

Acknowledgement

This chapter is an output of research commissioned and funded by the Policy Research Programme in the Department of Health, UK. The views expressed are not necessarily those of the Department.

Further reading

Benoit, C., *et al.* (2005). Community-academic research on hard-to-reach populations: benefits and challenges. *Qualitative Health Research, 15*, 263–82.

Liamputtong, P. (2007). *Researching the vulnerable.* London: Sage.

Nind, M. (2009). *Conducting qualitative research with people with learning, communication and other disabilities: Methodological challenges.* ESRC National Centre for Research Methods Review Paper. (National Centre for Research Methods.) Available at: <http://eprints.soton.ac.uk/65065/1/MethodsReviewPaperNCRM-012.pdf> (accessed 10 September 2012).

Rugkasa, J. and Canvin, K. (2011). Researching mental health in minority ethnic communities: reflections on recruitment. *Qualitative Health Research, 21*, 132–43.

Walmsley, J. (2004). Inclusive learning disability research: the (nondisabled) researcher's role. *British Journal of Learning Disabilities, 32*, 65–71.

References

Aldridge, J. (2007). Picture this: the use of participatory photographic research methods with people with learning disabilities. *Disability and Society, 22*, 1–17.

Atkinson, R. and Flint, J. (2001). Accessing hidden and hard-to-reach populations: snowball research strategies. *Social Research Update, 33*, 1–4.

Beadle-Brown, J., *et al.* (2012). *Engagement of people with long term conditions in health and social care research: Barriers and facilitators to capturing the views of seldom-heard populations.* Working paper 2849. UK: QORU.

Begum, N. (2005). *Doing it for themselves: Participation and black and minority ethnic service users.* London: Social Care institute for Excellence. Available at: <http://www.scie.org.uk/publications/reports/report14.pdf> (accessed April 2012).

Booth, T. and Booth, W. (1994). Use of depth interviewing with vulnerable subjects. *Social Science & Medicine, 39*, 415–24.

Cabinet Office. (2010). *Inclusion health: Improving the way we meet the primary health care needs of the socially excluded.* London: HMSO. Available at: <http://cabinetoffice.gov.uk/social_exclusion_task_force/short_studies.aspx>.

Cameron, L. and Murphy, J. (2007). Obtaining consent to participate in research: the issues involved in including people with a range of learning and communication disabilities. *British Journal of Learning Disabilities, 35*, 113–20.

Department of Health. (2010). *Inclusion health: Improving primary care for socially excluded people.* London: Department of Health. Available at: <http://www.dh.gov.uk/prod_consum_dh/groups/dh_digitalassets/@dh/@en/@ps/documents/digitalasset/dh_114365.pdf>.

Dickson-Swift, V. (2005). *Undertaking sensitive health research: The experience of researchers.* Unpublished doctoral thesis, Department of Public Health, School of Health and Environment, La Trobe University, Bendigo, Australia.

Emmell, N. and Clark, A. (2009). *The methods used in connected lives: Investigating networks, neighbourhoods and communities.* ESRC National Centre for Research Methods, NCRM Working Paper Series 06/09. Available at: <http://eprints.ncrm.ac.uk/800/>.

Garland, J., Spalek, B., and Chakraborti, N. (2006). Hearing lost voices: issues in researching 'hidden' minority ethnic communities. *British Journal of Criminology, 46*, 423–37.

Goodley, D.A. (2000). *Self-advocacy in the lives of people with learning difficulties: The politics of resilience.* Buckingham: Open University Press.

Howard, L., *et al.* (2009). Why is recruitment to trials difficult? An investigation into recruitment difficulties in an RCT of supported employment in patients with severe mental illness. *Contemporary Clinical Trials, 30*, 40–6.

Hyden, L.C and Brockmeier, J. (2008). *Health, illness and culture; Broken narratives.* London: Routledge.

Keen, S. and Todres, L. (2007). Strategies for disseminating qualitative research findings: three exemplars. Forum: Qualitative Social Research, *8*(3), Art. 17.

Kittay, E. (1999). *Love's labour: Essays on women, equality and dependency.* New York, NY: Routledge.

Lloyd, V., Gatherer, A., and Kalsy, S. (2006). Conducting qualitative interview research with people with expressive language difficulties. *Qualitative Health Research, 16*, 1386–404.

Lu, Y., Trout, S.K., and Creswell, J.W. (2005). The needs of AIDS-infected individuals in rural China. *Qualitative Health Research, 15,* 1149–63.

McCall, L. (2005). The complexity of intersectionality. *Signs, 30,* 1771–800.

McCormack, M., Adams, A., and Anderson, E. (2012). Taking to the streets: the benefits of spontaneous methodological innovation in participant recruitment. Qualitative Research. First published online 27 July. Available at: <http://qrj.sagepub.com/content/early/2012/07/27/1468794112451038>.

Martinez-Ebers, V. (1997). Using monetary incentives with hard-to-reach populations in panel surveys. *International Journal of Public Opinion Research, 9,* 77–87.

Meadows, L.M., *et al.* (2003). Balancing culture, ethics and methods in qualitative health research with Aboriginal peoples. International Journal of Qualitative Methods, *2*(4), Art. 1. Available at: <http://www.ualberta.ca/~iiqm/backissues/2_4/pdf/meadowsetal.pdf>.

Mental Capacity Act 2005. (2005). London: HMSO.

Morris, S.M. (2001). Joint and individual interviewing in the context of cancer. *Qualitative Health Research, 11,* 553–67.

Morrow, E., *et al.* (2012). *Handbook of service user involvement in nursing and healthcare research.* West Sussex: Wiley-Blackwell.

Morse, J.M. (2002). Interviewing the ill. In Gubrium, J.F. and Holstein, J.A. (eds) *Handbook of interview research: Context and method,* pp. 317–28. Thousand Oaks, CA: Sage.

Murphy, J. and Cameron, L. (2005). *Talking mats: A resource to enhance communication.* Stirling: University of Stirling.

Nelson, H.L. (2001). *Damaged identities, narrative repair.* Ithaca, NY: Cornell University Press.

Oliver-Africano, P., *et al.* (2010). Overcoming the barriers experienced in conducting a medication trial in adults with aggressive challenging behaviour and intellectual disabilities. *Journal of Intellectual Disability Research, 54,* 17–25.

Steel, R. (2005). Actively involving marginalised and vulnerable people in research. In Lowes, L. and Hulatt, I. (eds) *Involving service users in health and social care research.* London: Routledge.

Thompson, S. and Phillips, D. (2007). Reaching and engaging hard-to-reach populations with a high proportion of nonassociative members. *Qualitative Health Research, 17,* 1292–303.

Tuffrey-Wijne, I., Bernal, J., and Hollins, S. (2008). Doing research on people with learning disabilities, cancer and dying: ethics, possibilities and pitfalls. *British Journal of Learning Disabilities, 36,* 185–90.

Walmsley, J. (2001). Normalisation emancipatory research and inclusive research in learning disability. *Disability and Society, 16,* 187–205.

Chapter 14

Participatory action research: using experience-based co-design to improve the quality of healthcare services

Glenn Robert

This chapter explores the origins and development of an intervention—experience-based co-design (EBCD)—that is designed to capture, understand, and improve patients' experiences, before going on to provide an overview of a typical implementation and reflecting on the evidence base for such approaches. Possible future developments in the field of co-design and other 'dialogic' forms of organizational development are then discussed. The chapter begins by setting efforts to improve patients' experiences in the broader context of the 'quality movement' in healthcare.

Using patients' experiences to improve the quality of healthcare services: a brief history

Healthcare policy frameworks in several countries describe 'patient experience' as a core component of healthcare quality, alongside clinical effectiveness and patient safety (see, for example, Department of Health (2010)). Nonetheless, patient experience has commonly been perceived as the softest of these three components and the one to which less attention has been paid over the last 15 years of the 'quality movement'. As Robert and Cornwell (2011) have argued, measuring patient experience has lagged behind the development of indicators of clinical effectiveness and patient safety, at least in terms of investment and sophistication.

The development of frameworks to define and understand patients' experiences of healthcare can be traced to at least the early 1990s. As Coulter describes (Chapter 2), both the Institute of Medicine and Picker frameworks—the best known, technically sound, and most useful of a plethora of attempts to define and categorize what matters to patients—originate in research by Gerteis et al. (1993) in the USA. More recently, Iles (2011, p. 36) distinguishes between *transactional* aspects of care—a set of 'efficient auditable transactions between consumers and providers'—and the *relational* aspect of care—'a covenant between care giver and care receiver…that recognises that neither is an impersonal unit in a care transaction…but a whole richly multifaceted person whose physical responses are strongly bound to emotional ones'. She highlights the dangers of not taking into account both these aspects when seeking to understand and improve patients' experiences. I return to this observation later in this chapter.

There is no shortage of general recommendations to healthcare organizations as to how to capture patient feedback and use it to improve patient experience, see for example, Coulter et al. (2009) and National Health Service (NHS) Confederation (2010). In addition, there are various reviews focusing on specific aspects or challenges relating to patient feedback, for example, on the use of real-time feedback technologies (Brown et al., 2009), and developments in the area of outcome measures for chronic conditions (National Centre for Health Outcomes Development, 2006). Since the late 1990s there has been a corresponding step change in how healthcare organizations collect, share, and reflect on patients' experiences but still little systematic and responsive improvement work goes on at the coalface to actually improve this important component of the quality of healthcare services.

Internationally, healthcare organizations tend to use questionnaire surveys to provide patients' perspectives on how they are performing. In England, acute hospital trusts are increasingly deploying a wider range of methods and approaches locally. Yet, there is evidence that local clinical teams and middle management make little use of national patient survey data to monitor service quality and drive local quality improvement. As Robert and Cornwell (2011, p. 9) conclude, 'current measures of patient experience are not being used meaningfully or systematically at the local level for a range of reasons but, not least, because they are not seen as clinically relevant at a service level, and are captured too infrequently'.

Large-scale surveys across multiple organizations can play an important role in meeting broader policy agendas such as accountability and transparency. Much has been achieved through the rigorous development and sustained commitment to surveying patient views of their experiences. Yet surveys may be less effective at supporting local quality improvement if they lack clinical credibility, are insufficiently timely or specific to guide action by senior leaders (see Chapter 9). These issues have been major barriers to patient experience being placed on an equal footing with clinical effectiveness and patient safety as a key dimension of healthcare quality (Robert and Cornwell, 2011).

Different methods of collecting patient experience data can also produce different results. As this volume illustrates, all methods have their strengths and weaknesses and organizations which rely solely on survey data may overlook important nuances of how patients reflect on their care experiences. To illustrate, an elderly lady completed both a patient survey and a narrative interview exploring her experiences on an acute elderly care ward (Maben et al., 2012); in her response to the survey question 'Overall, did you feel you were treated with respect and dignity while you were in hospital?', she ticked the box 'Yes, always'; similarly, in response to the survey question 'Overall, how do you rate the care you received?', she ticked the box 'Excellent'. And yet the following is an extract from her narrative interview:

> The other thing I didn't raise and I should have done because it does annoy me intensely, the time you have to wait for a bedpan…elderly people can't wait, if we want a bedpan it's because we need it now. I just said to one of them, 'I need a bedpan please'. And it was so long bringing it out it was too late. It's a very embarrassing subject, although they don't make anything of it, they just say, 'Oh well, it can't be helped if you're not well'. And I thought, 'Well, if only you'd brought the bedpan you wouldn't have to strip the bed and I wouldn't be so embarrassed'.

The contrasting quality improvement implications arising from these different methods of capturing this experience could not be starker. The results from the patient survey would not lead to any action, indeed the ward team could be commended for the excellent, dignified care it provided, whereas the narrative interview revealed how annoyed and embarrassed the lady was as a result of an interaction that had clearly formed a lasting impression of her subjective experience.

So, given the shortcomings of existing (largely quantitative) methods, where should we look for alternative approaches that might hold the key to understanding and improving the relational aspects of patient experience? The focus of this chapter is on enabling change at the local level through the use of a quality improvement intervention with the explicit aim of improving patients' experiences.

Experience-based co-design: the origins and influences

I will discuss in turn the four, overlapping, strands of thought that have contributed to the development of the EBCD approach, namely:

♦ participatory action research
♦ user-centred design

- learning theory
- narrative-based approaches to change.

With its roots in social psychology and phenomenology and important influences from the likes of Kurt Lewin and Paolo Freire, participatory action research (PAR) sets out—in contrast to a traditional, positivist, science paradigm—to recognize and directly address complex human and social problems. Although encompassing a wide range of research practices, McIntyre (2008, p. 1) proposes four underlying tenets to the majority of PAR projects:

(a) a collective commitment to investigate an issue or problem, (b) a desire to engage in self- and collective reflection to gain clarity about the issue under investigation, (c) a joint desire to engage in individual and/or collective action that leads to a useful solution that benefits the people involved, and (d) the building of alliances between researchers and participants in the planning, implementation and dissemination of the research process.

Action research has not had a particularly distinguished record in the healthcare sector, or indeed in other policy areas. Much of the early action research in healthcare was criticized for poor design and lack of rigor, and it was often neither educative nor empowering for those involved. Proponents of PAR have since argued that the sacrifice of some methodological and technical rigor is worth the additional face validity and practical significance that is gained.

With similar roots to PAR, user-centred (or participatory) design draws its inspiration from a subfield of the design sciences (which include architecture and software engineering) whose distinctive features are: (a) direct user and provider participation in a face-to-face collaborative venture to co-design services, and (b) a focus on designing experiences as opposed to systems or processes. Ethnographic methods such as observation and narrative interviews (see Chapters 3 and 5) are thus preferred. User-centred design makes two particular contributions to quality improvement thinking. Firstly, it offers a new lens, or frame of mind, through which to conceive approaches to improving patients' experiences of healthcare; primarily its pragmatic nature highlights the importance of 'making sense' of experience and finding solutions to poorly designed interactions. Secondly, it offers methods, tools, and techniques (such as modelling and prototyping) which were little used in healthcare improvement work until very recently.

The influence of learning theory on the development of EBCD emerges from a wide variety of sources including Argyris and Schön (1978), and more recently Kerr and Lloyd (2008), Wheatley (2009), and Kerr (2010). The central argument is that, in contrast to traditional forms of management and clinical skills training, we should be training 'reflective practitioners', enabling staff to 'draw back', to pause, reflect, and gather information, people, and insight. The implications for improving patient experiences of healthcare services are that we should: (a) focus on what both groups (staff and patients) want, and (b) provide a 'safe haven' within which to rehearse and practise new ways of thinking, feeling, doing, and relating. Emotional disclosure in which discussion of emotions is constructed as a normal and healthy human activity is an important part of this (Howard et al., 2000; Drew, 2008).

Finally, narrative approaches are an important strand because 'stories and storytelling are the basis of EBCD ... [they] contain huge amounts of information, wisdom and intelligence about experiences that are waiting to be tapped as a rich source for future service development and design' (Bate and Robert, 2007a, pp. 66–7). In keeping with PAR, user-centred design and learning theory, narrative-based approaches to change are premised on subjective, socially constructed stories that enable connections with 'assumptions, values, expectations, cognitions and emotions' (Bate and Robert, 2007a, p. 65).

Taken together, these four strands of thought also relate to the increasing interest in what Bushe has termed 'dialogic' organizational development (OD) approaches (Bate and Robert, 2007b). Such approaches have turned away from traditional, top-down, leader-centric, and diagnosis-led OD and towards practices that 'assume organisations are socially co-constructed realities' and have in common 'a search for ways to promote dialogue and conversation more effectively' as it is 'by changing ... conversations that normally take place in organisations that organisations are ultimately transformed' (Bushe, 2009, pp. 619–20).

The experience-based co-design approach

Shaped by these four strands, and first piloted in 2006/07 in a head and neck cancer service in the south of England (Bate and Robert, 2007a), the resulting EBCD approach has now been implemented in breast and lung cancer pathways across two large London teaching hospitals in the UK (Tsianakas et al., 2012), several emergency departments in New South Wales, Australia (Iedema et al., 2010), and numerous other NHS settings in England and Scotland (Hodgkiss et al., 2011). An EBCD 'toolkit' has been developed and is freely available online (The King's Fund, 2012). Ongoing research is exploring the spread and sustainability of the approach as well as an adaptation designed to 'accelerate' its implementation and impact. A full description of the EBCD approach is given elsewhere, accompanied by a case study of the pilot implementation in a head and neck cancer service (Bate and Robert, 2007a).

Figure 14.1 details the six stages of the action research process that together make up the EBCD approach to improving patient experiences. Stage 1 involves establishing the governance and project management arrangements. The fieldwork underpinning an EBCD project typically then begins with a four-month data collection period (stages 2 and 3). In stage 2, a wide variety of staff (from, for example, receptionists to lead clinicians) are interviewed about their experience of working within a service using a semi-structured interview schedule; over multiple implementations of the approach we have found that the data from approximately 12 to 15 interviews provide sufficient insights for the purposes of being able to represent back and reflect on staff experiences. The staff interviews are transcribed and analysed thematically. Non-participant observation helps to contextualize and understand patient experiences from both the patient and staff perspective; for example, in a recent EBCD project two researchers conducted a total of 219 hours of participant observation of clinical areas along the relevant patient pathway

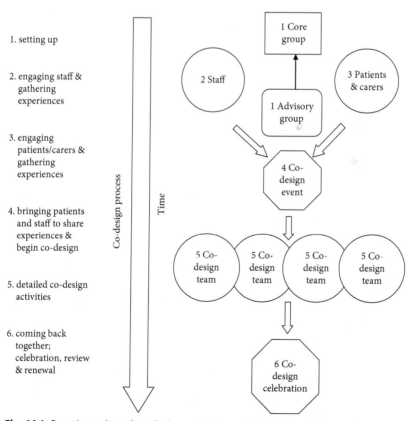

Fig. 14.1 Experience-based co-design: a six-stage design process.

(Tsianakas et al., 2012). The specific aspects of care that are observed are not pre-determined and the observations focus on both functional and relational aspects of patient/staff interactions. Following the data collection, staff met to review the themes arising from the staff interviews and observational data in order to identify their priorities for improving services (see Figure 14.1).

In stage 3—which runs in parallel with stage 2—patients and carers are recruited (for example, through clinical nurse specialists in outpatient clinics) and an experienced qualitative researcher conducts filmed, narrative-based, unstructured interviews lasting, on average, one hour, in which patients describe their experiences of care since first diagnosis. Each patient is then sent their own film to view before deciding whether it can be shared with other patients and staff. Two researchers view the films independently to ensure analytical rigour and shared understanding of significant 'touchpoints' (Dewar et al., 2010). 'Touchpoints' are the crucial moments, good and bad, that shape a patient's overall experience; the concept originated in the airline industry and represent the key moments where people's subjective experience of the service is shaped. Exemplar 'touchpoint moments' that emerged from the pilot implementation of EBCD in a head and neck cancer service included: breaking of the bad news; percutaneous endoscopic gastrostomy (PEG) feeding tube; 'waking up in an Intensive Care Unit'; the cancer ward; 'looking in the mirror'; and radiotherapy and radiotherapy planning.

Films are then edited to produce one composite 35-minute film, representing all the key touchpoints in a service. In addition, audio recordings of the narrative interviews can be transcribed and the data analysed thematically. All the patients and carers are invited to a showing of the composite film, following which a facilitated group discussion highlights any different or emerging issues. An emotional mapping exercise is then used to help patients reflect together on the emotional impact of the touch points (Bate and Robert, 2007a, p. 128). Following this group work, patients vote on their shared priorities for improving services.

In stage 4 the respective staff and patient priorities are presented at a joint event at which staff view the composite patient film for the first time. Mixed groups of patients and staff use the issues highlighted in the film, together with the priorities from the separate staff and patient meetings, as a basis to identify joint priorities for improving services. Patients and a variety of medical, allied health professional, and administrative staff then volunteer to join specific 'co-design working groups' (typically four to six groups) to design and implement improvements to services (stage 5), initially over a three-month period. The majority of these groups are facilitated by quality improvement specialists from the participating healthcare organization and ground rules are established from the outset, ensuring all participants have equal voices.

At stage 6, these separate co-design working groups reconvene to discuss their work to date and plan the next stages of the improvement process.

Evaluation findings

There is growing evidence that EBCD can bring about changes which improve patient experience, and are acceptable to a range of service users. For example, an independent evaluation of EBCD in three emergency departments in New South Wales, Australia, found that it had led to significant improvements, changes in practice, and learnings for clinical and health departmental staff, as well as engaging consumers in 'deliberative' processes that were qualitatively different from conventional consultation and feedback (Iedema et al., 2008; Piper and Iedema, 2010). The researchers commented that, 'on a broader front, co-design has been shown to strengthen service provider-service user relationships...co-design harbours a collaborative principle that should be woven into how health services and health departments conceptualise and structure their communication with patients, families and the public'. In England, Farr (2011) found that as well as making specific changes to various aspects of breast and lung cancer services, the project also supported wider improvements, including helping to establish a wider culture of patient involvement, and facilitating greater and more open team working and better communication across departments, clinicians, and staff of different grades (see Figure 14.2).

Strengths and limitations

Several evaluations highlight the central importance played by key 'brokers' and facilitators of such patient-centred improvement work and of ongoing organizational support. Expert brokering is necessary both for implementing approaches like EBCD locally as well as for disseminating such approaches beyond isolated 'islands of improvement'. Also crucial to the success of approaches like EBCD are the discursive, narrative-based interactions between staff and patients that are enabled by the change process (Iedema et al., 2010). The filmed patient narratives are key in triggering these interactions and fulfil several functions: they are a tool for reflective learning (for both patients and staff); they provide data to drive the co-design process; and they (re-) establish an emotional connection between the staff and patients. In the following quotation a staff member considers the impact of watching the patient film:

> for me this is about 'Oh God, they're our patients aren't they?' when people watch the film they might think, 'I remember that lady', they know they're our patients—they can't get away from the fact—but it actually makes it more real for them. Whatever

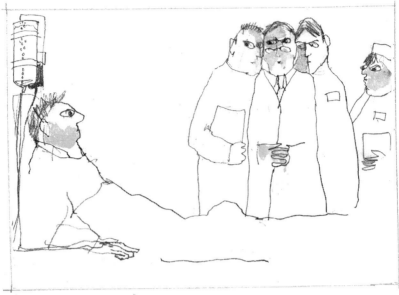

the ward round

Fig. 14.2 'The ward round'. Reproduced with kind permission from Nick Wadley, *Man + Doctor*, Dalkey Archive Press, London, UK, Copyright© 2012 Nick Wadley.

way they're captured, it's about capturing it so that people recognise these are patients I have cared for, nursed, met, who are saying this...and I think that's what is so different from other improvement work in terms of things like discovery interviews and focus groups: it's that direct connection between them.

EBCD has therefore been found to result in improved service quality, but one of the major barriers to widespread implementation is the time and cost involved in the discovery phase (stages 2 and 3 in Figure 14.1). Replicating five to six months of qualitative interviewing and non-participant observation on each patient pathway in a healthcare organization may be considered impractical. Adaptations of the approach are therefore in development and being piloted with the aim of 'scaling up' the benefits of EBCD more efficiently across different settings. 'Accelerated' approaches may not work as well if, for example, local staff and patient engagement in the change process is less forthcoming. However, even if 'accelerated' forms of EBCD do not work as well as the traditional approach, they may work 'well enough' to be worth pursuing.

The direction of travel

Integral to the EBCD approach is that patient, carer, and staff experiences are used systematically to co-design and improve services. As such, EBCD is part of a much broader movement around co-production and co-design in public services. It is also aligned with the work of 'revisioning' OD as described by Bushe and Marshak (2009), with a 'focus on exploring common aspirations and the design of preferred futures as key outcomes of the change process'.

So where to next in the search for ways to capture, understand, and improve patients' experiences in healthcare organization? The current 'research into practice' agenda looks a little like this:

◆ Consolidating what we have learnt in different organizational contexts about (a) successful implementation (in particular the crucial role of facilitators), and (b) spread and sustainability.

◆ Testing new ('accelerated') forms of co-design approaches that better suit practitioner needs.

◆ Employing EBCD as part of a broader, multilevel OD intervention.

◆ Methods and approaches for capturing, understanding, and improving staff experiences alongside patient experiences (and exploring links between the two).

◆ Further theorizing about 'co-design' in healthcare and its implications for (a) service redesign, (b) improving the relational aspects of patient care, and (c) changing behaviours and mindsets in organizations.

Further reading

Bate, S.P. and Robert, G. (2007a). *Bringing user experience to health care improvement: The concepts, methods and practices of experience-based design.* Oxford: Radcliffe Publishing.

Bate, S.P. and Robert, G. (2007b). Towards more user-centric organisational development: lessons from a case study of experience-based design. *Journal of Applied Behavioural Science*, 43(1), 41–66.

Bushe, G.R. and Marshak, R.J. (2009). Revisioning organization development. Diagnosic and dialogic premises and patterns of practice. *Journal of Applied Behavioural Science*, 45(3), 348–68.

Iedema, R., *et al.* (2010). Co-design as discursive practice in emergency health services: the architecture of deliberation. *Journal of Applied Behavioural Science*, 46, 73–91.

The King's Fund. (2012). *Experience-based Co-design toolkit.* Available at: <http://www.kingsfund.org.uk/ebcd/> (accessed 28 May 2012).

References

Argyris, C. and Schön, D. (1978). *Organizational learning: A theory of action perspective.* Reading, MA: Addison Wesley.

Bate, S.P. and Robert, G. (2007a). *Bringing user experience to health care improvement: The concepts, methods and practices of experience-based design.* Oxford: Radcliffe Publishing.

Bate, S.P. and Robert, G. (2007b). Towards more user-centric organisational development: lessons from a case study of experience-based design. *Journal of Applied Behavioural Science, 43*(1), 41–66.

Brown, H., Davidson, D., and Ellins, J. (2009). *NHS West Midlands Investing for Health Realtime Patient Feedback Project. Final report.* Birmingham: Health Services Management Centre, University of Birmingham.

Bushe, G.R. (2009). Dialogic OD: turning away from diagnosis. In: Rothwell, W.J., *et al.* (eds) *Practicing organization development: A guide for managing and leading change* (3rd edn), pp. 617–23. San Francisco, CA: Pfeiffer- Wiley.

Bushe, G.R., and Marshak, R.J. (2009). Revisioning organization development. Diagnostic and dialogic premises and patterns of practice. *Journal of Applied Behavioural Science, 45*(3), 348–68.

Coulter, A., Fitzpatrick, R., and Cornwell, J. (2009). *Measures of patients' experience in hospital: Purpose, methods and uses.* London: The King's Fund.

Department of Health. (2010). *Liberating the NHS: Transparency in outcomes. A framework for the NHS.* London: Department of Health. Available at: <http://www.dh.gov.uk/en/Publicationsandstatistics/Publications/>.

Dewar, B., *et al.* (2010). Use of emotional touchpoints as a method of tapping into the experience of receiving compassionate care in a hospital setting. *Journal of Research in Nursing, 15* (1), 29–41.

Drew, G. (2008). An artful learning framework for organisations. *Journal of Management & Organization, 14,* 504–20.

Farr, M. (2011). *Evaluation report of the patient centred care project.* London: King's Fund. Available at: <http://www.kingsfund.org.uk/publications/articles/patient-centred-care-project-evaluation-report>.

Gerteis, M., *et al.* (1993). *Through the patient's eyes: Understanding and promoting patient-centered care.* San Francisco, CA: Jossey-Bass.

Hodgkiss, F., Barrie, K., and Sinclair, C. (2011). *Better together. Experience based design cancer pilots. Interim reflection report.* March 2011. Available at: <http://www.knowledge.scot.nhs.uk/media/CLT/ResourceUploads/1008115/EBD%20CancerPilots%20InterimReflection%20Report%20Version1.0.pdf>.

Howard, C., Tuffin, K., and Stephens, C. (2000). Unspeakable emotion: a discursive analysis of police talk about reactions to trauma. *Journal of Language and Social Psychology, 19,* 295–314.

Iedema, R., *et al.* (2008). *Emergency department co-design stage 1 evaluation—Report to health services performance improvement branch, NSW Health.* Sydney: Centre for Health Communication, University of Technology Sydney.

Iedema, R., *et al.* (2010). Co-design as discursive practice in emergency health services: the architecture of deliberation. *Journal of Applied Behavioural Science, 46,* 73–91.

Iles, V. (2011). *Why reforming the NHS doesn't work. The importance of understanding how good people offer bad care.* Really Learning. [Online] Available at: <http://www.reallylearning.com/Free_Resources/MakingStrategyWork/reforming.pdf>.

Kerr, C. (2010). Community engagement and artful academic staff development: a return on expectations through collaborative practice. *International Journal of Work Organisation and Emotion, 3*(4), 384–99.

Kerr, C. and Lloyd, C. (2008). Pedagogical learnings for management education: developing creativity and innovation. *Journal of Management and Organization, 14*(5), 486–503.

McIntyre, A. (2008). *Participatory action research*. Thousand Oaks, CA: Sage.

Maben, J., *et al.* (2012). "Poppets and Parcels": the links between staff experience of work and acutely ill older peoples' experience of hospital care. *International Journal of Older Peoples Nursing, 7*, 83–94.

NHS Confederation. (2010). *Feeling better? Improving patient experience in hospital*. London: The NHS Confederation.

National Centre for Health Outcomes Development. (2006). *A structured review of patient-reported measures in relation to selected chronic conditions, perceptions of quality of care and carer impact*. Report to the Department of Health. Oxford: National Centre for Health Outcomes Development.

Piper, D., and Iedema, R. (2010). *Emergency department co-design program 1 stage 2 evaluation report*. Sydney: Centre for Health Communication (UTS) and NSW Health (Health Service Performance Improvement Branch).

Robert, G., and Cornwell, J. (2011). *'What matters to patients'? Policy recommendations. A report for the Department of Health and NHS Institute for Innovation & Improvement*. Warwick: NHS Institute for Innovation & Improvement.

Tsianakas, V., *et al.* (2012). Implementing patient centred cancer care: using experience-based co-design to improve patient experience in breast and lung cancer services. *Journal of Supportive Care in Cancer, 20*(11), 2639–47.

Wheatley, M. (2009). *Turning to one another: Simple conversations to restore hope to the future*. San Francisco, CA: Berret-Koehler Publishers.

Chapter 15

Understanding and using health experiences: the policy landscape

Bob Gann

Patient empowerment is here to stay. Healthcare systems throughout the world have recognized that patient experience is an incomparably rich resource. If we are serious about improving the quality of care provided, we need to listen to the voice of patients, analyse what patients are telling us, and respond with service change. As the 2012 World Health Organization conference on patient empowerment argued, there needs to be a global shift away from the traditional paternalistic approach to healthcare that ignores personal preferences and creates dependency, to a patient-centred approach. 'Indeed in countries such as China and India, health systems will only cope with the onslaught of chronic disease with patient empowerment' (Anon., 2012).

Policy context: international

Patient involvement has become increasingly central to health policy in many countries in recent years. Policymakers are aware that the active engagement of patients in their own care holds the key to strengthening self-care, choosing appropriate and effective treatments, improving health outcomes driving service improvement, and ultimately delivering affordable and sustainable services (Coulter, 2011).

The European Commission recognizes the importance of patient involvement within health policy in its White Paper *Together for Health: A Strategic Approach for the EU 2008-2013*. In 1992, Finland passed the world's first patients' rights legislation and this has been followed by countries including Belgium, Cyprus, Denmark, France, Netherlands, Slovenia, and Spain. During the 1990s, several countries (including Austria, Germany, Ireland, Malta, Sweden, and the UK nations of England, Wales, and Scotland) developed Patients' Charters which highlighted patient rights. Patient engagement and involvement has consistently been a key plank of system reform, highlighted in health plans including the Labour government's National Health Service (NHS) Plan in England and the Italian National Health Plan (Harter et al., 2011).

The emphasis on patient empowerment is not just a European but a world-wide phenomenon. The Canadian Patients' Bill of Rights and the Public Patients Hospital Charter in Australia both include the right to partici-pate fully in healthcare decisions. In the USA, President Obama's *Patient Protection & Affordable Care Act* incorporates a Patients' Bill of Rights, although focusing specifically on consumer protection and choice within health insurance.

Policy context: United Kingdom

Angela Coulter has traced the origins of patient empowerment to the 1960s counter-culture, and subsequent policy developments. In the UK, successive governments have embraced patient activism from both community and con-sumerist perspectives. This focus has continued with the Conservative–Liberal Democrat coalition elected in 2010. The key recent legislation in England is the *Health and Social Care Act 2012*, which builds on themes of public empow-erment, choice, and service transparency which has been consistent through governments of different political persuasion over recent years. The Act states the duty of the Secretary of State to secure continuous improvement in the quality of services including 'the quality of experience undergone by patients'. It establishes bodies including HealthWatch with responsibility for listening to 'the views of people who use health or social care services on their needs and experiences', and the NHS Commissioning Board which has a duty to promote 'the involvement of each patient, carer and representative in deci-sions relating to their care and treatment'. The NHS Commissioning Board has a wide range of powers and functions, including 'to engage with the public, patients and carers, champion patient interests and ensure patients have access to a wide range of information about services'.

The themes in the new Act had been signalled in the White Paper *Equity and Excellence: Liberating the NHS* (Department of Health, 2010) which was pub-lished soon after the Conservative–Liberal Democrat coalition government came into office. *Liberating the NHS was* aimed at putting patients and the public at the centre of health care. The White Paper promised an 'information revolution' to ensure patients are equipped to exercise greater choice and con-trol, including enabling patients to rate the quality of care they receive in hospi-tals and clinical departments. *Liberating the NHS* anticipated a cultural shift to shared decision-making being the norm: 'no decision about me without me'.

Policy levers

So how do we make patient engagement a reality? Governments have a range of levers, command and control measures (legislation, regulation, performance targets, and financial incentives), good practice guidelines, and pressure from public and patients' expectations.

In England, *The Operating Framework for the NHS 2012/13* (Department of Health, 2011) sets out the planning, performance, and financial requirements for which NHS organizations are held to account. Putting patients at the centre of decision-making is one of the four key themes of the 2012–13 framework, with a weight equal to maintaining a grip on finances, increasing productivity and quality, and completing transition to the new health and care system and structures. Key objectives are to ensure patients have a positive experience of care, and to help patients and the public to understand how the NHS is performing in relation to patients' outcomes. The framework says bluntly 'Each patient's experience is the arbiter of everything the NHS does'.

To support the commitment to improve experiences of NHS care, evidence-based 'how to' guides, and examples of good practice have been assembled (NHS Institute for Innovation and Improvement, 2012). Research commissioned from the Kings Fund and Kings College London (Robert and Cornwell, 2011), and the Picker Institute's Principles of Patient Centred Care have informed the National Quality Board's framework for patient experience (Department of Health, 2012a). It outlines those elements that are critical to experience of NHS services. The National Institute for Health and Clinical Excellence (NICE) has published patient experience quality standards—one for mental health (NICE, 2011a) and one for adult services (NICE, 2011b), which describe what high-quality patient experience looks like and how it might be measured in these service areas.

In addition to frameworks and guidelines, hard payments can be used to incentivize improvements in patient experience. The Commissioning for Quality and Innovation payment framework enables commissioners to reward excellence by linking provider income to achievement of local quality improvement goals, including patient experience.

Healthcare policy has consistently seen information for patients and the public as an enabler for supporting patient autonomy and control, increasing choice, and driving service improvements through greater transparency. The Department of Health's information strategy *The power of information: Putting us in control of the health and care information we need* (Department of Health, 2012b) makes a firm commitment to providing much richer information on performance, quality, and experience of care. This will range from outcomes data (including patient reported outcome measures, see Chapter 8) and clinical audits through to feedback, comments, and stories from staff and patients. Every encounter with health and care services is an opportunity to collect views and experiences of patients and carers through technologies that will include online SMS and bedside television. An increase in the volume of routine feedback, wherever possible in real time at the point of care, is encouraged. From 2013, patients leaving hospital will be asked 'Would you recommend this service to your friends and family?'. However it should be noted that real-time feedback may produce more 'socially desirable reporting' from patients who may be feeling grateful or vulnerable (see Chapter 9).

Throughout these policies it is useful to distinguish between the linked but distinct themes of voice and choice:

+ Voice—information gathered from patients through feedback, surveys, ratings, and comments to drive quality improvement.

+ Choice—information (including the experience of others) provided to patients to help them decide between treatment options and healthcare providers.

Voice: capturing and acting on patient experience

The inquiry into poor standards of care at two hospitals in central England, graphically illustrated that the NHS has not always been ready to listen to the experience of patients (Mid-Staffordshire NHS Foundation Trust Inquiry, 2010). The Parliamentary and Health Service Ombudsman's report *Listening and Learning* (2011) described an inconsistent, at times unacceptable, approach by some NHS organizations to handling complaints: 'NHS organisations must actively seek out, respond positively, and improve services in line with patient feedback'. The results from regular surveys of patients (Chapter 9), staff, and service users are published on the NHS Choices website. Taken together these provide a picture of the quality of patient experience, which can be enhanced by in-depth qualitative studies (Chapters 3–7)

In addition to structured surveys of patients' experience, there is an increasing range of user-generated information. As Mazanderani and Powell describe in Chapter 10, more formal, solicited routes for capturing patient experience are increasingly dwarfed by the scale of spontaneous sharing through online blogs, forums, communities, and social networks of people—an incredibly rich, and as yet largely untapped, resource for understanding patient experience

User comment on products and services is a common phenomenon. Many online shoppers and consumers today read and post comments and ratings on sites such as Amazon (<http//www.amazon.co.uk>), eBay (<http//www.ebay.co.uk>), TripAdvisor (<http//www.tripadvisor.co.uk>), and Top Table (<http//www.toptable.com>) which all invite customer reviews. The consumer feedback aggregation and syndication service Reevoo (<http//www.reevoo.com>) displays over 500 million consumer reviews to 120 retailer, publisher, and manufacturer websites. Increasingly, user ratings and comments on public services including health and social care are appearing. These may be moderated before publication and may include the opportunity for services to respond.

A Pew Internet national survey of 3,000 respondents in the USA (Fox, 2009) found:

- 41% of e- patients (those who are online and have used for health information) have read someone else's commentary of their experience of a health issue.
- 24% of e-patients have consulted online rankings or reviews of hospitals or other providers.
- 24% of e-patients have consulted online rankings or reviews of doctors or other professionals.

However, although reading experiences is very common, far fewer actively contribute their own experience:

- 6% of e-patients have posted a comment on online forum.
- 5% have posted comment about a doctor.
- 4% have posted a comment about a hospital.

In addition to ratings and comments, there are also a large number of online communities, enabling user-generated comment and networking between people with shared experiences, conditions, or problems. The Pew study also found 20% of e-patients have accessed an online health community or social network, and one in four Internet users living with a chronic condition have gone online to find others with similar health concerns.

Choice: information to support decisions on treatment and care

Reflecting these modern realities, several countries have established online information portals to provide people with information to support choice, both of healthcare provider and treatment options. National portals in the Netherlands (<http://www.kiesbeter.nl>), Denmark (<http://www.sundhed.dk>), and Sweden (<http://www.vardguiden.se>) provide information for the public on healthy lifestyles, self-care for common conditions, treatments, and services available. The Sundhed portal is particularly well developed, providing access to networks of patients with similar diagnoses, personal health data within the health record, and online appointment bookings, prescription renewals, and communication with health professional. In the USA, the Affordable Care Act led to the establishment of the US government's HospitalCompare site (<http://www.hospitalcompare.hhs.gov>) where patients can compare providers by a range of comparative indicators, including patient experience captured through the national HCAHPS survey (Hospital Consumer Assessment of Healthcare Providers and Systems).

In England, the government-funded national portal NHS Choices (<http//www.nhs.uk>), established in 2007, receives over 15 million visits a month in 2012. NHS Choices is most commonly used for information on conditions and treatments, and finding services, although there is also content on healthy lifestyles. Patient comment and ratings have been an integral part of the service from the start. Over 80,000 comments have been published to date. Users can rate services against a series of closed questions (including a net-promoter question 'Would you recommend this service'), and can also leave free text reviews. All comments are pre-moderated before publication; providers are alerted so they can post a response.

The leading independent comment service Patient Opinion (<http//www.patientopinion.org.uk>) was established in 2005 by a Sheffield general practitioner, Dr Paul Hodgkin, as a not-for-profit social enterprise. Patient Opinion emphasizes the conversation between users and health services. Rather than encouraging criticism of healthcare staff, which can be one-way and unproductive, Patient Opinion invites comments which can be tracked on the website to see what has happened to the progress of the story, who has read it, and what action has been taken (Hodgkin, 2010).

Services like NHS Choices and Patient Opinion allow patients to report their experiences of a hospital service, general practice, etc. but not of an individual clinician. Opposition from professional bodies, legal risks of defamation, and quite proper concerns about protecting staff from abuse, mean that identification of individuals is moderated out before publication. However, accounts of experience at hospital level can be a blunt instrument. Quality of care, culture, and communication can vary considerably across departments and clinical teams. The independent comments and ratings service iWantGreatCare (<http//www.iwantgreatcare.com>), established by Dr Neil Bacon, an

Oxford nephrologist, has tackled this head-on through a service which enables patients to rate individual clinicians.

The opportunity to comment on individuals without 'moderation' is more extensive than is often realized. It is easy for anyone to set up a comment website and for patients worldwide to post ratings of their clinician. The US doctor rating site, RateMDs (<http//www.ratemds.com>) has over one million ratings of individual clinicians, including UK doctors.

Despite these developments, the volume of comment posted remains very small compared with the numbers of contacts: NHS Choices receives up to 200 patient comments a day in a national health service which has over a million patient contacts a day. Online forums and communities enable user-generated comment and networking between people with shared experiences, conditions, or problems. These often provide invaluable insights into people's experiences of using services, but often in a less structured way. There are thousands of online communities for specific issues, including rare conditions, where the online environment offers the opportunity to meet others with the same condition regardless of geography.

In addition to issue-specific communities there are also umbrella communities such as HealthUnlocked in the UK (<http://www.healthunlocked.com/>) and PatientsLikeMe in the USA (<http://www.patientslikeme.com/>) which provide access to communities and individuals with wide range of conditions. PatientsLikeMe represents a new but growing development in shared patient experience—shared use of what is often considered private information: personal health data (Wicks et al., 2010). The model is of a central repository for all personal health information generated within clinical contexts (e.g. health history, diagnosis, current treatments, medication) kept securely for view by patients and their healthcare providers, but also shared with 'patients like me' by offering the ability to search for other similar users by criteria including symptoms, treatments, and demographics (Frost and Massagli, 2008). Although the funding model is made explicit on the PatientsLikeMe site, the approach has attracted some controversy because revenue is based on selling aggregated data to organizations including pharmaceutical companies.

These communities can be seen as part of the phenomenon of the patient centred approach to pharmacovigilance described by Anderson and Herxheimer in Chapter 12. Although patients have the opportunity to report adverse drug reactions formally through the yellow card reporting system, far greater numbers are sharing their experiences of medicines spontaneously through online communities.

Emerging policy themes

As we move into an era of 'no decision about me without me' a number of emerging information policy themes are being debated.

Shared decision-making

The government wants shared decision-making to be the norm in the NHS. As well as being an ethical imperative, there is compelling evidence that patients who are active partners in their own care have better outcomes than patients who are passive recipients of care (Coulter and Collins, 2011). Shared decision-making is particularly important for preference sensitive decisions, where there may be several feasible treatment options so personal priorities, invisible to the clinician, are therefore key. Here it can be particularly helpful for patients to hear and see the experiences of other patients and the decisions they made (for example, through HealthTalkOnline, <http://www.healthtalkonline.org>) or to use patient decision aids such as those commissioned under the Quality Improvement Productivity and Prevention Right Care Shared Decision Making Programme led by NHS Midlands and East.

However, despite the policy commitment, there is still some way to go towards shared decision-making being the norm. There is now the opportunity for the NHS Commissioning Board, in its role as champion of patient and carer involvement, to play a key part. The Health Foundation has set out critical steps for the NHS Commissioning Board to make 'no decision about me without me' a reality. Participants in a Health Foundation summit (Health Foundation, 2012) called on the Board to:

- Engage in the development of a strong narrative for shared decision making.
- Inspire others to play their part.
- Invest in the development of robust and meaningful measures of patients' involvement in their own care.
- Proactively encourage changes in service provision.

The role of the state

The UK government is committed to increasing opportunities for patients to provide feedback and share their experiences. But such services do not necessarily have to be provided by governments. Some people will undoubtedly want to give their views directly to the NHS; others will prefer an independent route. This may particularly be the case where their experience of care has led to a loss of confidence and trust in the NHS.

The *Power of Information* (Department of Health, 2012b) strategy suggests that there are political, social, and economic reasons for the state to step back from some areas of information provision, and to look to independent information organizations, including patient groups and social enterprises, for innovation. 'A number of organisations already enable us to provide online feedback about our care, and others are coming into the market. Central government will not seek to duplicate this specific function but will look to pool comments made on external sites on a national portal. In return this will help to stimulate new traffic to those sites to help them become sustainable' (Department of Health, 2012b, p. 69).

Quality and risk in patient experience

Reading and listening to the experiences of other patients can be empowering and supportive, but there are undoubtedly risks. As has long been observed (White and Dorman, 2001) online communities, comment and ratings services, and patient experiences websites can create opportunities for mistaken, inaccurate, or dangerous medical advice. Social networks can be open to abuse by 'trolls' (people who post derogatory comments under a cloak of anonymity). There are two main approaches to ensuring quality and minimizing risk: moderation and adoption of quality standards. Responsible comments sites pre-moderate postings before publication to remove comments which are libellous, abusive, racist, etc. It is a more difficult judgement to moderate comments which are passionate, aggressive, or intemperate. They may still be trying to tell us something important about the experience of care received.

Conscious of the highly variable quality of online health information, a number of quality accreditation schemes have been established. The Health on the Net Foundation launched its voluntary certification scheme in 1996. Run by a not-for-profit foundation based in Geneva it has certified websites in over 100 countries as meeting the standards of the HON Code (<http://www.hon.ch>). In England, the Department of Health has sponsored the Information Standard (<http://www.theinformationstandard.org>), an independent voluntary scheme which accredits providers of good quality providers of health information. HealthTalkOnline was one of the first organizations to gain Information Standard certification, because of the quality of its information development processes and the evidence base of its work. There remains a need to reconcile the sometimes conflicting benefits of listening to the authentic voice of patients (which may be less structured and more emotional).while at the same time protecting from harm, providing an appropriate level of quality assurance while avoiding an excessive level of intervention.

Validity of patient experience

Alongside concerns about potential harm from sharing patient experience, there is also the frequently expressed view that patient voice provides a less valid source of evidence, particularly when set aside harder data on quality of services. Sites such as Hospital Compare in USA and NHS Choices in England present a range of different quantitative and qualitative information side by side on comparative scorecards of healthcare providers. Patient stories sit alongside detailed directories of services and tables of clinical indicators covering infection, readmission, mortality, waiting times, etc. We need more research into this, but it is at least possible that when faced with an overwhelming amount of information a couple of vivid, engaging patient stories may carry disproportionate influence compared with more objective but less accessible data.

Healthcare providers have been very sensitive to this concern about the influence of subjective and possible atypical experiences (Lagu et al., 2010). However, some emerging research suggests that patient experience may be a good indicator of objective clinical service quality. Researchers at Imperial College London (Greaves et al., 2012) analysed patient comments on NHS Choices and Patient Opinion and compared these with clinical indicators for the same providers. They found there was a good correlation between patient views and quality data. Positive recommendations of hospitals were significantly associated with lower hospital standardized mortality ratios for high-risk (but not low-risk) conditions. Subjective assessments of hospital cleanliness matched lower MRSA (meticillin-resistant *Staphylococcus aureus*) and *Clostridium difficile* infection rates. Similarly, research analysis of patients' online ratings of their physicians over a five-year period in the USA (Gao et al., 2012) showed a good correlation between patient reviews of their doctor and measures of clinician quality including malpractice suits and recommendation by colleagues. It seems that despite professional scepticism, the crowd may indeed be wise (Surowiecki, 2004).

Looking forward: crowd sourced health services

In the second decade of the new millennium, we have unprecedented opportunities to listen to the experiences of patients: the stories they tell us of health, illness, and using health services. When channels of communication were less easy, people needed to be highly motivated to share their experience.

They tended only to do so if their experience was particularly bad or particularly good—or if their views had been actively solicited. Healthcare systems have traditionally been based on linear relationships between individuals and services, where information is provided one way to patients, rather than from patients and between patients. Now, particularly with the mass growth in social media, people can record and share their experiences simply and quickly, at no cost to healthcare systems. When comment is this easy it can become routine. Every day on Twitter people record small personal events which taken together can build a rich picture of the concerns of citizens and service users—locally, nationally, and across national boundaries. People are speaking: the challenge for healthcare policy and delivery is to listen, and to act to improve services.

Further reading

Coulter, A. (2011). *Engaging patients in healthcare*. Oxford: Oxford University Press.

Department of Health. (2012). *The power of information: Putting us in control of the health and care information we need*. London: Department of Health.

Gann, B. (2012). *Giving patients choice and control: Health informatics on the patient journey. IMIA Yearbook 2012*. Geneva: International Medical Informatics Association.

NHS Confederation. (2011). *Remote control: The patient practitioner relationship in a digital age*. London: NHS Confederation.

References

Anon. (2012). Patient empowerment: who empowers whom? *Lancet, 379*(9827), 1677.

Commission of the European Communities. (2007). *Together for health: A strategic approach for the EU 2008-2013*. White Paper. Brussels: Commission of the European Communities.

Coulter, A. (2011). *Engaging patients in healthcare*. Oxford: Oxford University Press.

Coulter, A. and Collins, A. (2011). *Making shared decision making a reality: No decision about me without me*. London: King's Fund.

Department of Health. (2010). *Equity and excellence: Liberating the NHS*. London: Department of Health.

Department of Health. (2011). *The operating framework for the NHS in England 2012/13*. London: Department of Health.

Department of Health. (2012b). *The power of information: Putting us in control of the health and care information we need*. London: Department of Health.

Department of Health. (2012a). *A framework for patient experience*. London: Department of Health.

Fox, S. (2009). *The social life of health information*. Washington, DC: Pew Research.

Frost, J.H. and Massagli, M.P. (2008). Social uses of personal health information within PatientsLikeMe, an online patient community: what can happen when patients have access to one another's data. *Journal of Medical Internet Research, 10*(3), e15.

Gao, G.G., *et al.* (2012). The changing landscape of physician quality reporting: analysis of patients' online ratings of their physicians over a 5-year period. *Journal of Medical Internet Research* 14(1), e38.

Gann, B. (2012). *Giving patients choice and control: Health informatics on the patient journey IMIA Yearbook 2012.* Geneva: International Medical Informatics Association.

Greaves, F., *et al.* (2012). Associations between web-based patient ratings and objective measures of hospital quality. *Archives of Internal Medicine, 172*, 435–6.

Harter, M., van der Weijden, T., and Elwyn, G. (eds) (2011). Policy and practice developments in the implementation of shared decision making: an international perspective. Theme issue. *Zeitschrift für Evidenz, Fortbildung und Qualität im Gesundheitswesen,* 105(4), 227–326.

Health and Social Care Act 2012. (2012). London: The Stationery Office.

Health Foundation. (2012). *Leading the way to shared decision making: the critical steps for the NHS Commissioning Board to make 'no decision about me without me' a reality.* London: Health Foundation.

Hodgkin, P. (2010). Big society or just big conversation? *Guardian Healthcare Network*, 28 July.

Lagu, T., *et al.* (2010). Patients' evaluations of healthcare providers in the era of social networking. *Journal of General Internal Medicine, 25*(9), 942–6.

Mid-Staffordshire NHS Foundation Trust Inquiry. (2010). *Independent inquiry into care provided by Mid-Staffordshire NHS Foundation Trust 2005–2009.* London: The Stationery Office.

NHS Institute for Innovation and Improvement. (2012). *Transforming patient experience: The essential guide.* Warwick: NHS Institute. Available at: <http://www.institute.nhs. uk/patient_experience/guide/home_page.html>.

NICE. (2011a). *Quality standard—service user experience in adult mental health.* London: National Institute for Health and Clinical Excellence. Available at: <http//www.nice. org.uk/guidance/qualitystandards/service-user-experience-in-adult-mental-health/ index.jsp>

NICE. (2011b). *Quality standard—patient experience in adult NHS services.* London: National Institute for Health and Clinical Excellence. Available at: <http//www.nice. org.uk/guidance/qualitystandards/patientexperience/home.jsp>.

Parliamentary and Health Service Ombudsman. (2011). *Listening and learning: The ombudsman's review of complaint handling by the NHS in England 2010–11.* London: Parliamentary and Health Service Ombudsman.

Robert, G. and Cornwell, J. (2011). *What matters to patients.* London: King's College and Kings Fund.

Surowiecki, J. (2004). *The wisdom of crowds.* New York, NY: Doubleday.

White, M. and Dorman, S. (2001). Receiving social support online: implications for health education. *Health Education Research, 16*(6), 693–707.

Wicks, P., *et al.* (2010). Sharing health data for better outcomes on PatientsLikeMe. *Journal of Medical Internet Research, 12*(2), e19.

Index

Note: Page numbers in *italics* refer to figures and tables.

Printed and bound by CPI Group (UK) Ltd, Croydon, CR0 4YY